Assessment Language and Cognitive Communication Difficulties in Dementia and Other Progressive Diseases

© 2013 J&R Press Ltd

All rights reserved. No part of this publication may be reproduced, stored in a retrieval system or transmitted in any form or by any means, electronic, mechanical, photocopying, recording, scanning or otherwise, except under the terms of the Copyright Designs and Patents Act 1988 or under the terms of a licence issued by the Copyright Licensing Agency Ltd, without the permission in writing of the Publisher. Requests to the Publisher should be addressed to J&R Press Ltd, Farley Heath Cottage, Albury, Guildford GU5 9EW, or emailed to rachael_jrpress@btinternet.com.

The use of general descriptive names, registered names, trademarks, etc. in this publication does not imply, even in the absence of a specific statement, that such names are exempt from the relevant protective laws and regulations and therefore free for general use.

Library of Congress Cataloguing in Publication Data
British Library Cataloguing in Publication Data
A catalogue record for this book is available from the British Library

Cover design: Jim Wilkie

Project management, typesetting and design: J&R Publishing Services Ltd, Guildford, Surrey, UK; www.jr-publishingservices.co.uk

Printed and bound by CPI Group (UK) Ltd, Croydon, CR0 4YY

Assessment and Therapy for Language and Cognitive Communication Difficulties in Dementia and Other Progressive Diseases

Anna Volkmer

J&R Press Ltd

Contents

Acknowledgements

1. **How can speech and language therapy services meet the needs of people with dementia?** 1
2. **Assessment** 19
3. **Treatment planning and goal setting** 59
4. **Therapy and management: Language impairment** 77
5. **Therapy and management: Cognitive communication difficulties** 109
6. **Therapy and management: Conversation partners** 141
7. **Decision making and capacity in dementia: Our role as speech and language therapists** 167
8. **Measuring outcomes of therapy** 197
9. **Finishing touches: Maintenance, review and discharge** 207

Afterword and useful contacts 217

Index 219

Acknowledgements

I would like to acknowledge Rachael Wilkie for giving me the confidence to try this; also my colleagues, both speech and language therapists and from other allied health disciplines, who provided support and advice. Finally, I'd like to thank my friends and family, particularly Jamie, Alba and my mother, who put up with me over the last year or so.

1 How can speech and language therapy services meet the needs of people with dementia?

Introduction

As our population ages, it changes. Different generations have different attitudes to health care. As time goes on, we also develop more evidence from research. In short, the public is now more informed and more assertive than ever before. People are able to search the Internet and access information on new or novel therapies, whether they are in clinical use or not. This means people are perhaps more able to ask for what they feel they need, rather than asking for clinical medical expertise on what they actually need. Either way, it seems to have become more acceptable to ask for help or treatment, and people with dementia are becoming increasingly proactive (Brodaty, 2006, cited by Taylor, Kingma, Croot & Nickels, 2009). Indeed, requesting a referral to speech and language therapy may be becoming more common.

These changes in attitudes and approaches are likely to be reflected in the increase in the number and type of referrals being made to speech and language therapy services for communication therapy. A recent study in New South Wales in Australia illustrated this. The study highlighted that the number of referrals made for people with primary progressive aphasia (PPA) to a local outpatient service had increased from nil to six per annum over the course of four years (Taylor et al., 2009). Similar services in the UK, such as the Queens Square outpatient services (De Vissier, 2012) and various services I have worked in have also reflected these changes. Indeed, I worked in one service that experienced a shift from having no referrals for people with PPA to the outpatient service to having seven referrals in one year. In fact, individuals with dementia represent the fastest growing clinical population served by speech and language therapists (Mahendra & Arkin, 2003). Yet clinicians remain anxious not to promote their services too much in this area to avoid being inundated, and then facing the dilemma of how to prioritize these patients.

This chapter discusses dementia in the 21st century: the incidence and projected increases in the number of people living with the disease. We will highlight how valuable these statistics are in estimating the number and types of patients who may experience communication difficulties. This chapter also provides an idea of how a speech and language therapy service can be structured to meet the needs of this client group. The remainder of this book will attempt to "demystify" therapy for people with dementia. It will focus on practical assessment, intervention planning and therapy approaches and how these tie in with current evidence-based practice.

Ageing and dementia: The statistics

Our population is ageing. The increase in the number of people who are living longer is resulting in a greater number of people in the community over the age of 65. An article published by the UK Office for National Statistics (Dunnell,

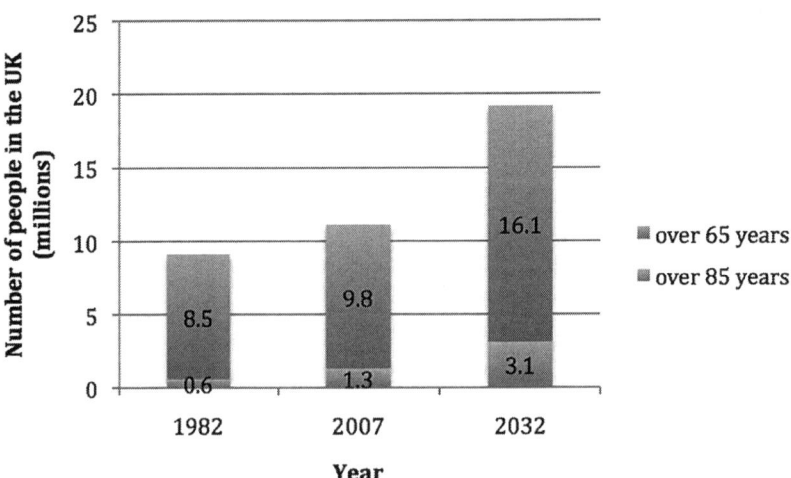

Figure 1.1 The recent and estimated increase in the number of people over 65 years of age living in the UK (data from Dunnell, 2008).

2008) stated that between 1982 and 2007 the number of people aged 65 years and over increased by 16% in the UK. The number of people over 85 years is projected to more than double by 2032 to make up 4% of the UK population. Together, people over 65 years of age will account for 23% of the total UK population by 2032. Figure 1.1 illustrates the estimated increase in the number of people over 65 years of age in the UK.

This information is significant for us as health care professionals working with older adults. Age is the single biggest risk factor for dementia. The increasing older population will inevitably have implications for the number of people living with dementia or at risk of developing dementia. Indeed, the Office for National Statistics projects that, by 2032, there may be around 1.4 million people living with dementia in the UK, double the number living with the disease at present. Worldwide figures report there are currently 36 million people living with dementia, and this is projected to increase to more than 115 million people by 2050 (Alzheimer's Disease International, 2008). Other researchers indicate a likely increase of 66% in the total number of people living with cognitive impairment between 1998 and 2031(Comas-Herrera, Wittenberg, Pickard, Knapp & MRC-CFAS, 2003). Yet it is not all doom and gloom; the increased numbers of people living with dementia also allow us to better understand the disease itself (Croot, 2009).

Dementia

It is valuable for every clinician to understand the impact that dementia has on our population. The gross statistics are as important as the smaller volume; both of these have implications for the numbers and proportions of patients we might expect on our clinical caseloads.

Dementia affects around 570,000 in England (National Health Service (NHS) website, 2012). Alzheimer's Disease International report that in the UK there are currently around 750,000 people living with dementia. They project that this figure will rise to over a million by 2021.

It is estimated that, at present, only 40% of people with dementia actually have a diagnosis (Alzheimer's Society website, 2012), suggesting that the reported incidence of dementia is significantly lower than what might be really happening. And from clinical experience this is something we are all aware of. There are often people who would rather not know, who are perhaps embarrassed or understandably afraid of these changes. More frustratingly, there are often patients who are well known to health services, who might not have a diagnosis, yet all those involved in that person's care know the individual has dementia. Everyone has the right to demand a specialist assessment and diagnosis from a qualified medical professional such as a consultant neurologist, geriatrician, psychiatrist or memory clinic service (NICE guidelines, 2011). As health professionals, we may sometimes take a role in supporting people to take this step if they would like to, or advocating for those who are no longer able to communicate this themselves.

The older an individual is, the greater the risk of dementia. The Alzheimer's Society and Alzheimer's Disease International estimate the incidence of dementia increases with the following pattern (see also Figure 1.2):

- in people over 65 years of age, 1 in 14 are living with dementia
- in people over 80 years of age, 1 in 6 are living with dementia
- in people over 90 years of age, 1 in 3 are living with dementia.

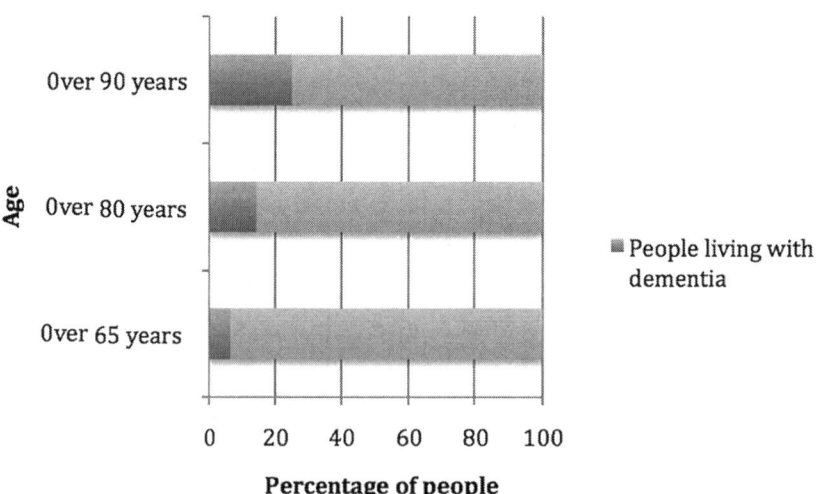

Figure 1.2 The estimated incidence of dementia (data from Alzheimer's Disease International).

It is important not to forget the people living with the younger onset variant of the disease. Even though the number of people under the age of 65 make up only a small percentage of the total number of people living with dementia they are still significant. The NHS UK website estimates that 2% of all dementias are diagnosed in people under the age of 65 years. The Alzheimer's Society reports that this numbers around 16,000 people currently in the UK. This is also valuable information for speech and language therapy services to be aware of: younger patients are more likely to have fewer co-occurring medical issues, have families, work and other social commitments. They are perhaps more likely to be 'generation X' type personalities who may demand more active treatments for their disease. More importantly perhaps for speech and language therapists, progressive aphasias are more likely to have a younger onset than other dementia variants.

The most common risk factor for dementia after age is gender. The majority of people living with dementia are also female. The Office for National Statistics reports that, at present, more females survive into older age than males. This suggests there is a larger cohort of people in the over 65s who are going to be more vulnerable to this disease simply because they are female. Indeed, Alzheimer's Disease International estimates that two-thirds of all people living with dementia are female.

The figures we have outlined here don't include everyone who is affected by dementia. We must not forget the numbers of partners, children and other family members or friends whose lives are affected by dementia. This disease will have a massive effect on all those living around the person who has been diagnosed with the disease. Caring for loved ones can have both a physical and an emotional impact on people's lifestyle, earnings and emotional status. So, not only do people with dementia lose communication skills, but people around the person will lose conversation partners and relationships.

The different variants of dementia

The large numbers described above can be even more relevant when they are broken down to reflect the different types of dementia. Different types of dementia have different neurophysiological presentations, different clinical characteristics and different patterns of progression. Understanding the prevalence of these different conditions can also allow us to understand the numbers of people who might be referred to us and why. Alzheimer's Disease

International has estimated the numbers of people living with different dementia types in terms of percentages (see Figure 1.3).

First and foremost, this list illustrates that the most common of all dementia variants is **Alzheimer's dementia**, accounting for approximately 465,000 people with dementia in the UK. This also suggests that the majority of people with dementia will probably develop memory difficulties that will affect conversation, and often word finding difficulties. These are all common features of Alzheimer's disease and are also reasons for a patient to be referred for speech and language therapy.

These statistics also highlight that of the 750,000 people living with dementia in the UK at present, at least 150,000 may be living with **vascular type dementia** or **mixed** vascular and Alzheimer's type dementia. Vascular dementia is often a consequence of a series of vascular events such as strokes, an area that speech and language therapists are comfortable that they are managing well. In these cases, we often find patients may have communication difficulties such as aphasia and dysarthria alongside the dementing disease. And in these cases, speech and language therapists may be pivotal in supporting conversation and communication through therapy tasks or adaptive strategies.

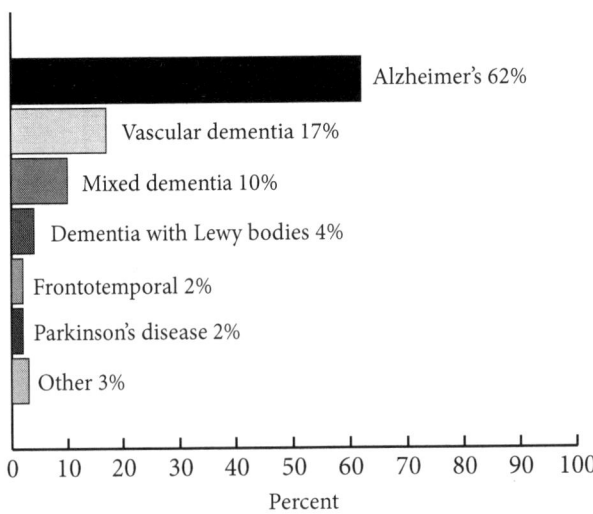

Figure 1.3 Breakdown of major variants of dementia (data from Alzheimer's Disease International, 2008).

Dementia with Lewy bodies affects around 300,00 people in the UK at present, according to these figures. This is another area of dementia where executive skills and communication may deteriorate very quickly.

This list also indicates that at present there are approximately 15,000 people living with a **frontotemporal variant of dementia** in the UK. Frontotemporal dementia can be subdivided into the behavioural variant or the language variant (primary progressive aphasias). Mesulam (2001) estimates that 20 percent of all people living with dementia have Primary Progressive Aphasia (PPA). This puts the number of people living with PPA in the UK at around 114,000, suggesting that there is a massive number of people with PPA or the behavioural variant of frontotemporal dementia who may be undiagnosed or misdiagnosed. There are three different types of Primary Progressive Aphasia: semantic, non-fluent/agrammatic and logopenic. As the names suggest, these variants of dementia are characterized predominantly by a language disorder, an area in which we are experts. This is also typically a younger onset variant of dementia. We know that the younger the client, the more likely they are to seek active treatment options such as speech and language therapy. This client group should be a group that speech and language therapists are involved with at the assessment as well as the therapy stage. We are able to provide expertise in differentiating between semantic, phonological and motor aspects of the communication impairment. And furthermore, evidence suggests that speech and language therapy treatment with this client group can significantly maintain language skills for a period of time.

Parkinson's disease is perhaps an area where we more commonly come across cognitive difficulties that make communication difficult. Around 15,000 people in the UK live with Parkinson's disease dementia. As therapists with an already well-established role in working with this patient group, we may see individuals repeatedly over a number of years dipping in and out of our services as their Parkinson's progresses. This allows us to monitor their communication and flag any changes in cognition such as attention to conversation and self-monitoring skills. We may be the first clinicians to become aware of cognitive decline in these individuals.

There are at least 22,500 people in the UK living with many **other variants** of dementia. Often these are people who are living with other conditions such as Motor Neurone Disease (MND), Multiple Sclerosis (MS), Progressive Supranuclear Palsy (PSP) and dementia in learning disability (such as Down's Syndrome) and who may cross our paths earlier in the disease process. There are also other less common conditions such as Huntington's disease, alcohol-related diseases such as Korsakof's dementia, Multiple Systems Atrophy (MSA) and Human Immunodeficiency Virus (HIV), which could all cause cognitive changes. People are living longer with these types of disease – they are being better physically managed. This means they are presenting with more complex cognitive issues, classified as dementia. The more we know, the more we can understand the likely clinical presentation and be prepared to deal with behaviours appropriately.

Most importantly, the figures outlined above tell us how many people could be referred to speech and language therapy. Who do these clients see if they do not see a speech and language therapist? As previously mentioned, there are many people who would prefer not to know, and occasionally someone who is aware of a diagnosis – such as Parkinson's disease – would prefer not to acknowledge that they are experiencing cognitive changes as part of the disease and only deal with the primarily physical issues. We must not forget these people are living with progressive diseases and sometimes they may have other priorities to deal with above and beyond the swallowing or the communication difficulties. But there are some who would like advice and support and it is for these people that we must endeavour to provide a more efficient and efficacious service.

The cost of dementia

To give you an idea of the amount of money that is potentially spent on this client group, the Office for National Statistics reports that currently around 40% of NHS funding is spent on those over 65 years of age according to a recent House of Commons committee report. McNamee, Bond and Buck (2001) estimated the formal health and social care costs associated with dementia in England and Wales at £0.95 billion for men and £5.35 billion for women in 1994, rising to an expected £2.35 billion for men and £11.20 billion for women with dementia in 2031 (based on 1994/95 prices). It is likely that the costs have risen even more since then.

However, the health service is not the only organization which is spending money on caring for people with dementia. Families spend money, forgo earning opportunities and lose investments to care for loved ones who become unwell. Social services spend money to assist people in everyday living, and charities attempt to fill gaps not covered elsewhere. At present, it is estimated that dementia costs the UK over £20 billion per year (Alzheimer's Society website).

Providing a speech and language therapy service for people with dementia

The National Institute for Health and Clinical Excellence and the Social Care Institute for Excellence produced a set of guidelines for supporting people with dementia, which they revised in 2011. This guideline states that "Communication is at the core of all effective psychological interventions, and communication strategies adapted to the individual's needs and abilities are the main building blocks to maximising skills and ensuring the least amount of dependency in care". In other words, speech and language therapists play an important role in caring for this client group, not just in the area of dysphagia management but also communication.

However, having stated that communication is a core aspect in managing all patients with dementia, there is no agreement in the clinical setting as to what speech and language therapy services should actually be providing for these patients. Various guidelines have been published advocating or recommending that speech and language therapy can be useful, but how and where is often not stated. On this note, Mahendra and Arkin (2003) have advocated that "speech and language therapists need to rethink, redefine and reclaim the spectrum of clinical services that they are qualified to provide to dementia patients".

In order to 'stake our claim' for speech and language therapy we need to consider the value of the care we can provide. Ultimately, outcomes are the health results that matter for a patient's condition over their episode of care. Two examples of this type of outcome might be a slower deterioration in the person's communication skills or increased functional independence and consequently less support required in their daily lives (Porter, 2009). What evidence do we have that suggests we can make a difference to people's health outcomes by providing a speech and language therapy service? Table 1.1 provides a summary of this evidence and illustrates in which settings investment in speech and language therapy services are currently best suited for people with dementia.

Table 1.1 Speech and language therapy services for communication in dementia.

Where should speech and language therapists see people with dementia for communication assessment and management?	What do the national clinical guidelines say?	What is the evidence for health outcomes?
Memory/dementia clinics *For assessment and diagnosis*	The NICE guidelines for dementia (2011) state very clearly that "Where there is also a significant impairment of language, an assessment by a speech and language therapist will contribute to the overall neuropsychological assessment. Such testing may provide important information regarding diagnosis and management".	Accurate diagnosis of dementia variants including the different PPAs assists in the identification of likely neuropathology and consequently allows a match to the most appropriate therapies as soon as possible (pharmacological or otherwise) (Croot, 2009; Bonner, Ash & Grossman, 2010; Dickerson, 2011).
Outpatients *For assessment, intervention and carer training*	The RCSLT (2009) state that treatment for people with dementia "should include intervention at an early stage based on communication strengths and weaknesses".	Evidence has demonstrated that the earlier an intervention can be given the more likely it is that we can maintain some aspects of communication through impairment-based therapies (see Chapter 4). And many patients are most likely mobile and living independently at home at this time. Indeed, there is evidence that this is when many people are increasingly asking for speech and language therapy interventions (Taylor et al., 2009).
Community *For assessment, intervention and carer training*		Research has demonstrated that treating people in their own environments better assists in carryover and maintenance of gains made in therapy (see Chapter 4). Being independent for longer costs less and provides better quality of life (Papp, Walsh & Snyder, 2009).

Psycho-geriatric or older adult	The National Service Framework for Older Adults states there should be a specialist old age multidisciplinary team, including speech and language therapists, as core members of that group in all general hospitals. They also state that specialist mental health services for older people should have agreed working referral arrangements with speech and language therapists.	At present it is estimated that 64% of people living in care homes have some type of dementia (Alzheimer's Society). Evidence has shown that training staff and carers in communication skills can significantly relieve the feeling of carer burden (see Chapter 6). Direct speech and language therapy has also been shown to reduce the incidence of agitated and difficult behaviours in residential settings (see Chapter 5).
Inpatient wards and nursing home/residential settings		
For carer training, assessment and intervention		

(NB: NICE: National Institute for Health and Clinical Excellence; PPA: Primary Progressive Aphasia; RCSLT: Royal College of Speech and Language Therapy.)

Having outlined where services may be best situated to manage communication difficulties in people with dementia, one cannot say they should not be seen or will not be seen in other settings. People with dementia may present on any clinical caseload; indeed, these are people who are likely to have multiple medical conditions, including dysphagia. However, patients with dementia who are admitted to acute general hospitals are unlikely to benefit significantly from support for communication at this time as the majority will present with severe deterioration in function due to a chest infection, urinary tract infection or cardiac concerns (Sampson, Blanchard, Jones et al., 2009). This suggests that the most useful advice from speech and language therapy at this time would be around swallowing. Patients with dementia are less commonly admitted to rehabilitation settings, and when they are it is likely that this is due to a separate event such as a stroke or fall. In these cases, it may be useful for speech and language therapists to understand the nature of the individual's communication needs and provide whatever support they can, but it is likely that other medical needs will take priority. Indeed, there is little evidence in the literature to support intervention for communication needs at these times.

Many speech and language therapy departments will have some type of service for people with dementia. Yet services have often been developed in an ad hoc manner and there will be many departments that will have little to no funding for this client group. Ponte (2000, cited by Ramsey, Heritage & Bryan, 2006) reports that in a survey of speech and language therapy services, around 67% of services in England see patients with dementia. Of these, 39% report that the service they do provide is quite casual. Any service planning to increase or set up a new service for people with dementia will have to consider many questions, including: who will manage this person operationally, will they fall into mental health services or not? Who will support their clinical supervision? And who will fund their training? Ramsey, Heritage and Bryan (2006) describe in detail many of the practical issues to consider in developing such a service.

However, in the first instance, adding another string to any department's bow requires resources. How do we apply for commissioning for this type of increase in resources? A starting point, suggest Ramsey et al. (2006), might be to identify and document the unmet needs in your speech and language therapy service for people with dementia. One way of doing this is to liaise with local stakeholders (people who might refer to you, or service users themselves) and ask them to complete questionnaires or participate in discussions to this effect. This baseline can then be used to measure the effectiveness of new services or provide a platform from which to request further resources. Linking this development of your service to national and local plans, as well as correlating it with data and demographics such as the percentage of older people in the area, or the incidence of dementia (as described above) can bolster your rationale (Ramsey et al., 2006).

Setting up a pilot project can be a good method of trialing a change and can demonstrate the value of further investment into such a service. Initial funding opportunities for such a project may not need to come from within the National Health Service. It might be helpful to apply for funding support from other sources such as charities and trusts. Such a project could aim to tackle specific areas of concern. As an example, could you trial the provision of training to nursing staff in a local dementia nursing home and demonstrate reductions in the number of agitated behaviours occurring, or demonstrate an improvement in the confidence of care staff? Can you alternatively demonstrate the added value that speech and language therapy assessment can provide to the assessment process for the team and patient in a memory or dementia clinic?

Commissioning challenges

The Department of Health in the UK released its White Paper titled 'Equality and Excellence: Liberating the NHS' in July 2010 in which they proposed a system of GP commissioning. This has dramatically changed the structure of the National Health system, and is something that we as a profession need to be mindful of when considering how to expand and maintain our services. Can we influence Central Commissioning Groups (CCGs) who will be advising the future commissioners on funding?

Part of these changes in the NHS will also impact upon education and training. Across England, Local Education and Training Boards (LETBs) will be set up as healthcare provider-led organizations and will be responsible for multiprofessional education and training arrangements. This means they will be assessing the requirements of local healthcare providers to develop training that helps staff meet the needs of the local population. In some areas, we may already be providing this type of training with nursing and care staff. Highlighting the effectiveness of this intervention to these new organizations can allow us to advocate for our role as trainers in communication skills for all staff members working with dementia. Perhaps joining forces with local branches of national organizations such as Dementia UK, the Alzheimer's Association and the Frontotemporal Dementia Support Group could also support your local status as an educator.

There will no doubt be further developments in these areas, and change is nothing new to the NHS. So consider perhaps that part of our role as a profession is to advocate for what we believe is best for our patients when change is afoot, and influence politics where possible to maximize services for our patients.

Providing evidence-based services to patients with dementia

Understanding and evaluating what is written in the research literature can be time consuming and difficult to access for the working clinician. Even though there has been growing recognition over the last 20 years that the work speech and language therapists do with this client group is worthwhile (Croot, 2009), few clinicians feel they really understand this themselves. A recent survey demonstrated that speech and language therapists in general practice did not necessarily feel confident in knowing how to manage the progressive aphasic client group, although they felt therapy was appropriate and in one case referred the client on to another speech and language therapy service for further support (Taylor et al., 2009).

Published research and studies on appropriate interventions for patients with dementia, particularly PPA, are only just beginning to appear in the speech and language therapy literature (Croot, 2009). The RCSLT (2009) states: "emerging practice will not have the same evidence base and therefore less empirically stringent measures of evidence need to be taken into account for these areas". This means that in areas such as dementia and speech and language therapy, where there is not a plethora of research, we will need to consider evidence from sources that are not necessarily 'the gold standard', i.e. randomized controlled trials.

The World Health Organization advocates that evidence-based practice does not just mean looking at published literature and research. We must listen to what experts in this area say and consult with the clients we are working with to develop our decisions. We can use written evidence – trials and descriptions of interventions – but also expert opinion such as that of published authors in the field. Indeed Croot (2009) suggests using psycholinguistic and learning theories to guide our practice with people with dementia, particularly progressive language impairment. Croot explains that psycholinguistic theories (which we are all familiar with from working with aphasic patients) allow us to make informed choices about how a treatment may work for individual clients, i.e. using assessment results to guide hypotheses and consequently treatment planning.

The final ingredient for evidence-based practice is being patient centered. Simply because the literature states something works does not mean it will work for everyone. People are not all the same, nor do we communicate in exactly the same way. Different aspects of communication may be more important for different people. By taking a patient-centered approach, seeking expert opinions and evaluating the literature we are able to tackle most problems that come up in clinical situations.

The remainder of this book aims to clear the fog around language and cognitive therapies for people with dementia, and provide practical advice on the day-to-day management of progressive communication difficulties. Each chapter will also highlight and summarize examples from the research literature to support clinical decision-making.

Summary

Understanding the bigger picture is valuable for every clinician working with patients with dementia. It enables us to plan for the future and focus our resources where they will be most valued and required. We know that the number of older adults in our society is increasing, and consequently that there are increasing numbers of people living with dementia. There is also an increasing awareness of our role as speech and language therapists working with these patients, particularly with specific groups such as those with primary progressive aphasias. Within departments, we need to advocate for our role with this client group in order to ensure the financial support we need to provide a service. Some evidence already demonstrates that speech and language therapy can maintain some specific language skills. We as a profession must take responsibility to try to contribute to this picture.

Alzheimer's Disease International is calling for improvements in dementia care skills. Hopefully, this book can support this movement by adding to the available resources for speech and language therapists in everyday clinical situations. This book aims to provide an update on some of the current evidence around assessing and managing dementia, and how this applies to a clinical setting. This is by no means a complete list, nor is it intended to be. This text aims to provide a summary and guide you in considering which approaches are available for management and where to look for more ideas.

References

Alzheimer's Disease International (2008) The prevalence of dementia worldwide. Downloaded from: http://www.alz.co.uk/adi/pdf/prevalence.pdf

Alzheimer's Society website (2012) Downloaded from: http://www.alzheimers.org.uk/dementiamap and http://www.alzheimers.org.uk/site/scripts/news_article.php?newsID=1164

Bonner, M.F., Ash, S. & Grossman, M. (2010) The new classification of primary progressive aphasia into semantic, logopenic or nonfluent/agrammatic variants. *Curr' Neurol Neurosci Rep.* 10 (6), 484–490.

Comas-Herrera, A., Wittenberg, R., Pickard, L., Knapp, M. & MRC-CFAS (2003) Cognitive Impairment in Older People: Its Implications for Future Demand for Services and Costs. Report to the Alzheimer's Research Trust, Discussion Paper 1728, PSSRU, LSE.

Croot, K. (2009) Progressive language impairments: Definitions, diagnoses, and prognoses. *Aphasiology* 23 (2), 302–326.

Department of Health (2001) National Service Framework for Older People. Downloaded from: http://www.dh.gov.uk/prod_consum_dh/groups/dh_digitalassets/@dh/@en/documents/digitalasset/dh_4071283.pdf

De Vissier, L. (2012) Primary Progressive Aphasia – an update. October 2012: SIG Psychiatry of Old Age Study Day (Southern UK).

Dickerson, B.C. (2011) Quantitating severity and progression in Primary Progressive Aphasia. *J Mol Neuroschi.* 45, 618–628.

Dunnell, K. (2008) Aging and mortality in the UK. National statistician's annual article on the population. Office for National Statistics.

Department of Health July 2010 Equity and Excellence: Liberating the NHS. Downloaded from: http://www.dh.gov.uk/prod_consum_dh/groups/dh_digitalassets/@dh/@en/@ps/documents/digitalasset/dh_117352.pdf

Mahendra, N. & Arkin, S. (2003) Effects of four years of exercise, language and social interventions on Alzheimer's Discourse. *Journal of Communication Disorders* 36, 395–422.

McNamee, P., Bond, J. Buck, D. & The Resource Implication Study of the Medical Research Council Cognitive Function and Ageing Study (2001) Costs of dementia in England and Wales in the 21st century. *The British Journal of Psychiatry* 179, 261–270.

Mesulam, M. (2001) Primary progressive aphasia. *Annals of Neurology* 49 (4), 425–432.

National Collaborating Centre for Mental Health commissioned by the Social Care Institute for Excellence National Institute for Health and Clinical Excellence (revised 2011) THE NICE -SCIE GUIDELINE ON SUPPORTING PEOPLE WITH DEMENTIA AND THEIR CARERS IN HEALTH AND SOCIAL CARE, National Clinical Practice Guideline Number 42 published by The British Psychological Society and Gaskell. Downloaded from: http://www.nice.org.uk/nicemedia/live/10998/30320/30320.pdf

National Health Service (NHS) website (2012) Downloaded from: http://www.nhs.uk/Conditions/Dementia/Pages/Introduction.aspx

Papp, K.V., Walsh, S.J. & Snyder, P.J. (2009) Immediate and delayed effects of cognitive interventions in healthy elderly: A review of current literature and future directions. *Alzheimer's Dementia* 5 (1), 50–60.

Porter, M.E. (2009) A strategy for health care reform – toward a value-based system. *The New England Journal of Medicine* 361 (12), 109–112.

Ramsey, V., Heritage, M. & Bryan, K. (2006) Developing speech and language therapy services in older age mental health. In Bryan, K. & Maxim, J. (Eds) *Communication Disability in the Dementias.* Whurr Publishers: London and Philadelphia.

Royal College of Speech and Language Therapists (2005a) Clinical Guidelines. Downloaded from: www.rcslt.org/resources/publications

Royal College of Speech and Language Therapists (2005b) Speech and language therapy provision for people with dementia. RCSLT Position Paper, RCSLT: London. Downloaded from: www.rcslt.org/resources/publications

Royal College of Speech and Language Therapists (2009) Resource Manual for Commissioning and Planning Services for SLCN Dementia. Downloaded from: www.rcslt.org/resources/publications

Sampson, E.L., Blanchard, M.R., Jones, L., Tookman, A. & King, M. (2009) Dementia in the acute hospital: Prospective cohort study of prevalence and mortality. *British Journal of Psychiatry* 195, 61–66.

Taylor, C., Kingma, R.M., Croot, K. & Nickels, L. (2009) Speech pathology services for primary progressive aphasia: Exploring and emerging area of practice. *Aphasiology* 23 (2), 161–174.

2 Assessment

Introduction

One of the most common comments I have heard from colleagues is that they fear trying to choose an assessment tool for patients with dementia, and are unsure about interpreting the information they gather. Yet we, as speech and language therapists, are experts in this type of assessment; indeed, we assess all our patients. Patients with dementia can be assessed in just the same way as any other patient group.

There are many approaches to assessing people with dementia, and generally speech and language therapists will consider not only the medical impairment, but also the person and their surroundings. The World Health Organisation's International Classification of Function Disability and Health (ICF) can be a useful framework to guide assessments (Threats, 2012). The concepts of impairment, activity and participation can support assessment, goal setting and intervention planning. The biopsychosocial model of dementia can also be a useful framework for assessing people with dementia. It considers the medical factors that affect the disease process as well as the psychosocial factors that can also influence how a patient presents and copes with their condition on a day-to-day basis. This model suggests that in both psychosocial and biological domains there are fixed factors (which relate to history or risk factors and therefore are not amenable to change), versus tractable factors (which may be amenable to change). Fixed factors include aspects such as education and IQ (psychosocial) as well as age (biological). All of these factors are unchangeable by the time the individual presents for therapy, and all influence the risk of dementia. Tractable factors include aspects such as reduced mental stimulation and social networks and support (psychosocial) as well as other medical problems such as urinary tract infections (biological). These are areas that are more likely to be influenced and changed. Using this model can support the development and identification of beneficial interventions, which are most likely to result in positive change (Spector & Orrell, 2010).

This chapter describes the features of language and cognitive communication deficit that speech and language therapists could expect to see in different types of dementia. It also discusses different approaches and available tools for assessment.

Assessing a patient with dementia

Some patients may be referred to speech and language therapy with a firm diagnosis in place, others may not. Some may not even have been told their specific diagnosis, although it has been documented. One survey found that up to 50% of patients referred to speech and language therapy had not been informed of their diagnosis of primary progressive aphasia (Taylor, Kingma, Croot, & Nickels, 2009). Alternatively, patients may present with multiple neurological disorders in their medical history (such as stroke and dementia). This means you will need to prioritize and analyze each area of difficulty differently (Shipley & McAfee, 2009). Whatever the case, is it is useful to have an understanding of how different dementia types typically affect cognitive and communication skills. This allows you to compare what you are told from the case history and referral with what you see. Understanding the different dementias also assists you in educating patients and their families, planning therapy and judging what might happen in your patient's future so you can prepare them appropriately.

Do not be afraid to challenge a diagnosis. Patients may have been referred to you with a tentative diagnosis which is yet to be confirmed. In other cases, you may find referrals come to you via pathways where a diagnosis has not yet been made. Whether they are inpatients, outpatients or in the community our assessment results can support the diagnosis that a neurologist, geriatrician, psychiatrist or other doctor might make. As speech and language therapists, our clinical observations are invaluable to this process. Our neuropsychology colleagues may be experts in assessing cognition, our medical colleagues may be experts in medical management, but we are experts in communication impairments. This includes cognitive impairment, language and speech. This is particularly true for conditions such as the primary progressive aphasias, which are differently diagnosed depending on speech and language breakdown.

Unfortunately, these different dementia diagnoses may at times be bewildering. So many different types of dementia and different classification systems have been developed in the last 20–30 years that it can become confusing (Croot, 2009). Many titles describe the clinical presentation (primary progressive aphasia), whilst others label the neuropathology (such as Pick's disease) assumed to be present (Croot, 2009). In clinical practice, however, it can be helpful to remember that, just as in stroke or brain injury, the patient's presentation reflects the area of the brain that has been directly affected or that is affected by a communicating region (Croot, 2009).

The following provides an overview of the major dementia subtypes that can appear on a speech and language therapy caseload, and which will be referred to throughout this text (particularly primary progressive aphasia and Alzheimer's dementia). I have included some other variants of dementia which (from personal experience) I have found clinicians find particularly complex. However, this is not an exhaustive list and there are many conditions on which I will not focus, such as MS and Huntington's disease, as there is much in the literature that can be found elsewhere. It is helpful to refer to texts and the literature to guide your understanding of these conditions, particularly as there is often new information to consider in this area. I would encourage you to remain abreast of these if you have the chance by referring not only to texts such as this one, but reading recently-published journal articles which can often provide the most up-to-date information. (Some of these can even be accessed for free via search engines such as pubmed.) Tables 2.1 and 2.2 also provide summaries of the primary progressive aphasias and all the dementias respectively.

Frontotemporal dementia

Frontotemporal dementia (FTD) refers to a range of non-Alzheimer's dementias caused by atrophy of the frontal and anterior temporal brain regions (Croot, 2009). There are two major categories of frontotemporal dementia: one involves progressive speech and/or language impairment, the other includes progressive changes in behaviour. The first of these is an umbrella category for the three primary progressive aphasia variants. It is worth being aware that, although the frontotemporal dementias are typically non-Alzheimer's type, there are some people who present clinically with symptoms consistent with FTD but who present with Alzheimer's pathology on autopsy. Refining the diagnostic processes is still a work in progress.

Although people with the behavioural variant of frontotemporal dementia will primarily demonstrate changes in behaviour, they do nevertheless present with severely impaired participation in communication and difficulties attending to and engaging with a conversational partner. These problems are attributable to their reduced interest in the environment and distractibility and have been summarized in the literature as difficulties in responding appropriately and in organizing discourse, poor self-monitoring and turn-taking, poor topic maintenance, and disordered prosody (Rousseaux, Seve, Vallet, et al., 2010).

Primary progressive aphasias

Primary progressive aphasia, or PPA, was first described by Pick and Serieux in the 1890s but was revisited in the more modern literature by Mesulam in the 1970s (Bonner, Ash, & Grossman, 2010; Gorno-Tempini, Hillis, Weintraub, et al., 2011). PPA currently describes a group of three subtypes of progressive language impairment associated with frontotemporal lobar degeneration (FTLD). Some professionals may classify these as a variant of frontotemporal dementia (FTD). The diagnosis of PPA requires that patients experience an insidious progressive deterioration primarily in language skills, with little changes in memory and other cognitive areas (Bonner et al., 2010). Communication is considered to be the only factor contributing to deterioration in activities of daily living (Croot, 2009).

PPA refers to a clinical presentation and not to a pathological cause, but it was generally thought that most cases would show frontotemporal lobar degeneration with inclusions immunoreactive to ubiquitin and TDP-43 (FTLD-TDP) (Bonner et al., 2010). However, recent research has shown that Alzheimer's-type pathology or frontotemporal lobar degeneration with tau-positive immunoreactivity (FTLD-tau) could be responsible for a significant number of these PPA cases (Bonner et al., 2010). Some reports suggest the most frequent cause of logopenic variant PPA is Alzheimer's disease (Gorno-Tempini, Brambati, Ginex, et al., 2008; Bonner et al., 2010). Consequently, many people diagnosed with lvPPA are now being considered as possible candidates for treatment with medications used with patients with Alzheimer's disease (Dickerson, 2011).

There are three variants of PPA: semantic dementia or semantic variant PPA, logopenic variant PPA, and non-fluent progressive aphasia or non-fluent/agrammatic variant PPA. These classifications are still quite recent in the literature and can be inconsistent across countries and academic institutions (Bonner et al., 2010). Some recent research has highlighted that PPA could be inherited in an autosomal dominant manner with mutations of the progranulin gene (Gorno-Tempini et al., 2011). Other genes have also been linked to FTLD and PPA (Gorno-Tempini et al., 2011). But generally PPA is considered a spontaneous disease.

It is really valuable to understand the presentation of these three variants so that identification and investigation of these patient groups can improve the appropriate therapy approaches adopted (Dickerson, 2011; Gorno-Tempini et al., 2011). Just as with any aphasic client, understanding their area of breakdown and preserved strengths allows the clinician to identify the appropriate therapy tasks and conversational strategies as well as establishing a clear performance baseline (Dickerson, 2011). Adopting a model such as the psycholinguistic framework can support you in making such distinctions (just as with any other aphasic client).

Semantic variant PPA

svPPA (or semantic dementia (SD) or semantic PPA (PPA-S) – resembles wernickes aphasia)

The main presenting pattern in the semantic variant PPA is a progressive deterioration in both expressive and receptive language skills. This is predominantly characterized by semantic impairment, particularly evident on naming, single word comprehension, verbal semantic category fluency tasks and non-verbal object knowledge and recognition. Less familiar objects and words are more impaired resulting in a frequency effect. Speech is relatively fluent and phonologically correct. Spontaneous speech is often empty, characterized by vague terms such as 'that' or 'thing' (Bonner et al., 2010). Kertesz, Jesso, Harciarek. et al. (2010) suggest that questioning of word meanings such as "What is television?" is the primary defining characteristic of svPPA. These patients also demonstrate reading difficulties (acquired surface dyslexia) such as reading words as they are spelt, for example 'broad' as 'brode'.

It is worth noting that the specific dysgraphias and dyslexias in neurodegenerative diseases are similar to those observed in non-progressive brain injuries (Papp, Walsh, & Snyder, 2009). This includes 'surface dyslexia and dysgraphia' which has been described in svPPA (difficulties with reading and spelling of familiar words with phonological plausible errors due to deficits in the orthographic lexicon) and 'phonological dyslexia and dysgraphia' which has been described in Alzheimer's disease, lvPPA and navPPA (difficulties in reading and spelling unfamiliar words using sounding-out methods due to deficits in the phonology-orthography conversion system) (Brambati, Ogar, Neuhaus, & Gorno-Tempini, 2009).

Patients with svPPA, however, demonstrate relatively spared grammar, phonology and number knowledge. In conversation, these patients will be able to stay on topic and expand the topic during a conversation at the mild stage of the disease, but their skills in topic maintenance and elaboration decline as the disease progresses (Wong, Anand, Chapman, et al., 2009).

It is worth noting that there is some disagreement in the literature on whether svPPA is a different condition to semantic dementia. Both conditions appear to present with similar language impairment, but in semantic dementia there appears to be an additional difficulty in visual recognition of objects and faces (Bonner et al., 2010). However, we will not make this distinction in this text.

FTD has been identified as the second most common neurodegenerative cause of dementia in the under 65s but svPPA may be more common in later life than previously assumed. svPPA may easily be misdiagnosed as Alzheimer's disease as patients often report 'loss of memory' as their main concern and they perform poorly on verbal episodic memory testing. However, patients with svPPA present with preserved day-to-day memory, episodic memory, orientation, visuo-spatial and perceptual skills.

On imaging, these patients present with cortical atrophy of the ventral and lateral anterior temporal lobe and the anterior hippocampus and amygdala in the left hemisphere (Croot, 2009; Bonner et al., 2010; Dickerson, 2011). The genetic influence in svPPA appears to be relatively low and it seems that svPPA is mostly sporadic. Survival rate in svPPA is variable (Hodges et al., 2009).

Logopenic variant PPA – lvPPA

Also known as logopenic progressive aphasia, progressive mixed aphasia and progressive conduction aphasia, this resembles global aphasia

This variant of PPA is characterized by slow speech with lots of pauses due to significant word-finding difficulties, but no agrammatism (Gorno-Tempini et al., 2011). Phonemic paraphasias are common in speech and naming but are different from the semantic variant, where patients frequently try to fill pauses with circumlocutions. It is also different from the non-fluent/agrammatic variant as articulatory deficits and agrammatism dominate for these patients (Gorno-Tempini et al., 2008). Consequently, the lvPPA patients fall into the 'fluent' category although they may appear slow and hesitant in conversation (Bonner et al., 2010).

Patients with logopenic variant PPA can repeat single words and digits accurately but demonstrate poor sentence repetition, digit span, word span and letter span. Similarly, they can understand single words accurately but present with sentence comprehension deficits. This is explained by a hypothesized deficit in the phonological loop or auditory short-term memory (Gorno-Tempini et al., 2008; Bonner et al., 2010). Significantly, they will present with relative sparing of motor speech (articulation), grammar, and single-word comprehension (Gorno-Tempini et al., 2008; Bonner et al., 2010).

lvPPA has been correlated with atrophy in the left caudal superior and posterior temporal and inferior parietal region on imaging (Gorno-Tempini et al., 2008; Bonner et al., 2010; Dickerson, 2011). There is an association between the neuropathology of patients with lvPPA and AD. Alzheimer's-type pathology may be responsible for a significant number of these cases. Indeed, compared to patients with the other PPA variants, patients with lvPPA tend to have poorer episodic memory, yet compared to patients with AD they still perform well on single-word comprehension and other semantic tasks (Bonner et al., 2010). However, as the disease progresses, single-word comprehension difficulties will also emerge (Bonner et al., 2010).

Nonfluent/agrammatic Variant PPA – navPPA

Also known as non-fluent progressive aphasia or progressive non-fluent aphasia, this resembles Brocas aphasia

This variant of PPA is characterized by dysfluent and effortful speech, with hesitations, retakes, and errors which often slow down the patient's rate of speech significantly. This has been attributed to an apraxia of speech and has been thought to contribute to the naming difficulties on assessment tasks. Patients with navPPA also produce less complex sentence structures and make frequent grammatical errors such as omitting determiners and failing to completely produce a subject–verb clause (Bonner et al., 2010). These patients also present with comprehension difficulties, particularly for complex grammatical phrases (Gorno-Tempini et al., 2011; Bonner et al., 2011).

Patients with navPPA are thought to present with an apraxia of speech. However, the presentation can also be attributed to phonological retrieval impairment. Errors are predominantly characterized by substitutions, insertions, deletions or transpositions rather than by ill-formed phonemes one would find in a motor impairment such as apraxia of speech (Bonner et al., 2010). Patients with navPPA present with communication quite similar to a Broca's aphasia, although these patients also present with executive difficulties which will progress till patients are practically mute (Bonner et al., 2010).

navPPA could also be easily mistaken for lvPPA due to the similarity in impaired repetition of phrases and sentences, speech sound errors and more spared single-word comprehension and object knowledge. However, patients with navPPA present with significant agrammatism and less impaired naming difficulties compared to patients with lvPPA (Bonner et al., 2010). This can easily be rated using a written assessment to reveal early grammatical errors (Gorno-Tempini et al., 2011).

Cortical atrophy in navPPA is localized to the anterior perisylvian region, then extends into the left prefrontal cortex (Dickerson, 2011) and left superior temporal cortex as well as posteriorly into the parietal lobe (Bonner et al., 2010). Atrophy of the left inferior frontal cortex has been found to correlate with impaired grammatical comprehension and consequently sentence processing in these patients (Bonner et al., 2010). It is now known that many patients with navPPA will progress to syndromes resembling the motor problems associated with cortico-basal syndrome or PSP, so eliminating any other limb and fine motor control difficulties in finger movements can assist in the differential diagnostic process (Gorno-Tempini et al., 2011).

Differential diagnosis

Differentiating between the three variants of PPA can be a significant challenge and not as straightforward as it first appears (see Table 2.1 for a summary and comparison of the three PPA variants), particularly as patients' symptoms change and evolve as the disease takes hold. This has led to many splits in the academic world about agreement on definitions of the subtypes. Bonner et al. (2010) suggest that these splits are potentially exacerbated by the differences in testing approaches across institutions. In general, the American model does not split PPA into three separate subtypes whilst the European model does (Croot, 2009).

The NICE guidelines (2011) propose two sets of diagnostic criteria for frontotemporal dementia:

- The Lund-Manchester criteria (Neary et al., 1998): The Lund-Manchester criteria recognizes three main syndromes: frontotemporal dementia, progressive nonfluent aphasia and semantic aphasia.

- The NINDS Work Group on frontotemporal dementia and Pick's disease (McKhann et al., 2001, cited by Croot, 2009): The NINDS Work Group criteria recognize two main presentations: frontal (behavioural) and temporal (language).

Neither set has, however, been prospectively validated against autopsy for people with PPA.

Previously, authors such as Mesulam (2001) suggested that in order to qualify for a diagnosis of PPA, patients needed to satisfy the criterion of two years of purely language decline without any other cognitive symptoms. This means some patients may go without a specific diagnosis for some time. Perhaps this is a little rigid. Croot (2009) suggests that as a patient's symptoms change there are three potential patterns of progression:

1. Selective decline in speech and/or language skills

2. Initial decline in language and/or speech with additional impairments arising as the disease progresses, such as behaviour or memory

3. Decline in language and/or speech alongside other deficits from the onset.

However, using recognized labels allows clinicians to communicate more effectively with one another on particular cases. Problems arise when different people use different terms, or use the same term to mean a different thing. It can be a very valuable experience for clinicians within a department to discuss what they all mean by particular terms, so that at least within a department you can all be sure you are speaking the same language.

The other important factor in identifying diagnostic categories using recognized standardized tests is that this identifies likely neuropathology and consequently allows a match to the most appropriate therapies (Croot, 2009; Bonner et al., 2010; Dickerson, 2011) as soon as possible (pharmacological or otherwise). There is some evidence that motor speech abnormalities appear to be stronger indicators of underlying tauopathies (Dickerson, 2011). But exact neuropathological diagnosis is difficult to complete prior to post-mortem examinations. It is carried out through the examination of a slice of brain tissue under a microscope, after it has been stained with a range of chemicals. This allows the atypical protein deposits (also called inclusions) to be seen. By examining the type, frequency and location of these protein deposits we can identify different neurodegenerative diseases. In PPA, it is mainly ubiquitin-positive inclusions, tauopathies or Alzheimer's-type neuropathology. svPPA is most likely associated with ubiquitin-positive inclusions or tauopathies, whilst lvPPA has been known to be associated with Alzheimer's-type neuropathologies and navPPA has been associated with tauopathies (Croot et al., 2009; Bonner et al., 2010).

These neuropathologies may also be linked with other diseases; for example, tauopathies are often present in movement disorders. There is some evidence that Motor Neurone Disease overlaps with the behavioural variant of FTD (Fletcher, 2012). It is thought that the proteins responsible for cell death have been found to be common across the two conditions, and that both will result in similar physical and cognitive impairments, albeit in a different sequence. However, although these conditions may share a common feature such as abnormal tau-protein collections; research has found that these formations differ somewhat in terms of their morphology and content (Zampieri & Difabio, 2006). The research in this area is relatively preliminary. However, as more and more treatments become available it will become more and more important to distinguish between underlying neuropathology as soon as possible (Croot, 2009; Bonner et al., 2010).

Other factors to consider for this client group

The age at onset of this disease and the duration of the illness appear to vary significantly. However, data reported in a number of longitudinal studies and summarized by Croot (2009) indicate that patients are often diagnosed with PPA in their late 50s or early 60s. The average length of life after symptom onset is around 7–10 years (depending on how early a diagnosis is made), with most people needing assistance with daily care tasks such as mobility and eating around a year prior to death. As with other dementia types, the most common cause of death is reported as aspiration pneumonia in this patient group (Croot, 2009; Dickerson, 2011).

However, prior to this there are many changes that can impact on people's daily lives other than the deterioration in communication. Perhaps some of the most distressing are the changes in behaviour, personality and social cognition. Depression, apathy and dis-inhibition have been reported as the most common areas of concern (McKhann et al., 2001, cited by Croot, 2009). These factors are particularly significant when planning therapy. We may find many of our patients are no longer interested in therapy as these other issues impact more on their lives. So understanding how your patient has been managing in these areas can also be valuable.

Table 2.1 Characteristics of the three PPA variants and the likely area of change on brain imaging.

Variant of PPA	Areas of impairment on assessment of communication	Areas of relative strength on assessment of communication	Likely area of change on brain imaging	Likely pathology
Semantic Variant PPA –svPPA (semantic dementia or semantic PPA)	Poor naming Poor word comprehension Poor object/concept understanding (frequency effect present) Surface dyslexia	Grammatically sound No speech disturbances Relatively fluent Accurate repetition	Anterior temporal	FTLD-TDP
Logopenic variant PPA – lvPPA (logopenic progressive aphasia or progressive mixed aphasia or progressive conduction aphasia)	Reduced sentence and digit span repetition Phonological errors – slow empty speech (phonological loop disorder) Impaired single word retrieval	Relatively unimpaired single word repetition and comprehension Grammatically sound	Left posterior temporo-parietal	AD/FTLD-TDP
Non-fluent/agrammatic variant PPA – navPPA (non-fluent progressive aphasia or progressive non-fluent aphasia)	Dysfluent Effortful, halting speech with speech sound errors (apraxia of speech) Agrammatic and simple sentence structures Difficulties understanding sentences	Relatively unimpaired single-word comprehension	Left posterior frontal and insular	FTLD – Tau

Alzheimer's dementia

Alzheimer's disease was first described by Alois Alzheimer in 1906 at a conference in Tubingen. Since then, dementia has been recognized as one of the most common diseases of ageing. Alzheimer's disease (AD) is a slowly progressive, degenerating disorder in which memory loss is the hallmark symptom (Bourgeois & Hickey, 2009). Although more than one cognitive area will be affected by the disease (Duncan & Siegal, 1998), loss of memory is the most commonly understood and typically the earliest symptom of the disease. The course of the disease varies between individuals, but generally Alzheimer's disease can be categorized into mild (up to 4 years in length), moderate (2–3 years in length) and severe (1–3 years in length) (Cotter, 2005). Cotter (2005) describes people with mild Alzheimer's disease as being generally independent with some difficulties in new learning and memory and perhaps a mild change in personality. As the individual becomes more moderately impaired they become more dependent and disorientated with more disorganized conversation and some psychotic symptoms or behaviours. Finally, at the severe and terminal stages of the disease they will be unable to walk or sit independently, be unable to recognize people or speak more than a few words and unable to focus on a task.

Communication in Alzheimer's disease is initially fluent with no articulatory, phonological or syntactic difficulties. Difficulties are associated with semantic impairment, which manifests itself initially as word-finding difficulties and progresses to affect use of abstract language and difficulties in comprehension of abstract and complex information (Bourgeois & Hickey, 2009). Reading, writing and pragmatics remain relatively preserved initially. However, as the semantic impairment progresses difficulties worsen and discourse becomes empty with increased use of stereotyped, automatic phrases and pronouns, e.g. he/she in place of names (Arkin et al., 2001). Reading also starts to become difficult whilst speech, phonology and syntax remain intact. In the later stage of the disease, however, communication becomes severely impaired with echolalic perseverative and unintelligible, non-meaningful utterances observed and eventually even mutism (Bourgeois et al., 2009).

Pragmatics can be more or less preserved in the mild-to-moderate stages of Alzheimer's disease in comparison with deteriorating lexical-semantic processing. This means that people present with relative preservation of comprehension of non-literal information, such as recognition of emotions in others. So social conversation can remain fairly unimpaired in the mild-to-moderate stages of the disease. However, by the moderate-to-severe stage, people with Alzheimer's disease will demonstrate increased difficulties in paying attention to their conversation partner. They will have difficulties in responding to open questions and presenting new information, reduced initiation or logically organizing conversation topics (Arkin et al., 2001; Wong, Anand, Chapman, et al., 2009). These difficulties will also impact on turn taking and topic maintenance (Rousseaux et al., 2010). This is related to increasing executive impairment. Yet other social skills, such as prosody, gaze, non-verbal feedback and gestures, will probably remain intact. However, it is always important to consider that the quality of a social interaction depends heavily on the skills of the conversation partner such that even a mildly impaired individual may struggle significantly if they are communicating with someone who is an unskilled communicator themselves (Rousseaux et al., 2010).

Psychiatric symptoms might also impact on the content of conversation of someone with Alzheimer's disease. Repetitive verbalisations of anxious, delusional and obsessive thoughts may be apparent earlier on. As the disease progresses the patient might demonstrate delusional ideas, hallucinations, personality changes, mood disorders and other behaviours (Bourgeois et al., 2009).

Alzheimer's disease primarily involves changes in the temporal and parietal lobes (Bourgeois et al., 2009). These changes are associated with the presence of amyloid plaques (only found in patients with Alzheimer's disease) and neurofibrillary tangles, which can be observed on biopsy in neuropathological examinations (Brak, Alafuzoff, Arzberger, Kretschmar & Tredici, 2006). Tau and amyloid proteins build up in the nerve cell bodies in the brain causing eventual cell death. This dead cell material is then converted to neurofibrillary tangles (Huber, Stuchbury, Burkle, Burnell & Munch, 2006). Amyloid plaques are aggregations of certain peptides which can activate inflammatory processes. This also results in cell damage and death (Huber et al., 2006).

Alzheimer's disease is most often sporadic but a small number has been linked to several genetic factors including mutations on chromosome 21, 1, 14 and 19 (Bourgeois et al, 2009). It is well recognized that a decline in language is a symptom of Alzheimer's dementia yet the literature on the pattern of language progression in Alzheimer's disease is fairly 'sparse' (Arkin & Mahendra, 2001).

Differential diagnosis

In general, patients with FTD demonstrate significantly greater loss of insight and awareness than patients with Alzheimer's' dementia (Salmon, Perani, Collette, Feyers, et al., 2007). However, loss of awareness is correlated with disease severity such that the more impaired, the less aware people are (Salmon et al., 2007). Patients with FTD demonstrate difficulties in behaviour and difficulties in communication as their primary areas of impairment, whereas patients with Alzheimer's disease demonstrate more significant memory difficulties as the predominant area of impairment (Salmon et al., 2007). Both FTD and Alzheimer's disease also demonstrate significant awareness of changes in affect (particularly depressive mood and irritability). These mood changes may be a consequence of the patient's awareness of their impairments. This combination can impact significantly on their participation in both therapy and everyday activities they previously enjoyed.

Vascular dementia

Vascular dementia can be caused by haemorrhagic or hypoxic ischemic cerebral brain lesions (strokes). It can also be caused by cerebro-vascular disorders and arteriosclerotic changes in the blood supply to the brain related to conditions such as hypertension, high cholesterol, diabetes, heart problems and some lifestyle factors (Alzheimer's society website, 2012).

Vascular dementia can result in cortical or sub-cortical changes. Sub-cortical lesions to the basal ganglia, thalamus and sub-cortical white matter are most common (Bourgeois et al., 2009). When there are predominantly ischemic changes in the sub-cortical white matter the condition can be labelled Binswanger's disease or small vessel disease, whilst multiple cortical and sub-cortical lesions are labelled multi-infarct dementia.

Vascular dementia is not only characterized by its sudden and stepwise onset and deterioration but is often accompanied by day-to-day fluctuations and gait changes, which are absent in Alzheimer's disease. People with vascular dementia may present with hemiparesis or physical symptoms commonly associated with stroke, or with reduced step length and height thought to be associated with changes in the sub-cortical white matter. Consequently, people with vascular dementia will also often present with aphasia, dysarthria and other speech and language difficulties associated with stroke. In contrast, individuals with Binswanger's disease (small vessel disease) will often present with primarily cognitive communication difficulties, particularly executive difficulties including lack of insight, apathy, delayed processing, reduced attention, fluctuating language skills (Bourgeois & Hickey, 2009), reduced facial expressions and speech difficulties (Alzheimer's society website, 2012).

Dementia with Lewy Bodies, Parkinson's dementia and PSP

Dementia with Lewy Bodies (DLB)

Dementia with Lewy Bodies is caused by small spherical protein deposits (named Lewy Bodies) in the neuronal cell bodies in the neocortex of the frontal and temporal lobes and basal ganglia. These interrupt the effect of acetylcholine and dopamine on brain functioning. Dementia with Lewy Bodies is characterized by its distinctive pattern of fluctuating cognitive, psychiatric and motor symptoms as well as the patient's sensitivity to antipsychotic medications (Neef & Walling, 2006).

Dementia with Lewy Bodies is often distinguished from Parkinson's disease by the occurrence of cognitive difficulties before or at the same time as the development of physical difficulties (Alzheimer's society website, 2012). This includes cognitive difficulties such as early attentional difficulties and hallucinations. However, many people with Dementia with Lewy Bodies will also present with symptoms of Parkinsonism such as rigidity, bradykinesia, tremor and gait abnormality (and postural change) (Bourgeois & Hickey, 2009). These symptoms of Parkinsonism may also affect speech and people will present with a flat affect, monotone dysphonic voice and dysarthria (Alzheimer's society website, 2012), In comparison to patients with Alzheimer's dementia, patients who present with Dementia with Lewy Bodies are more impaired on verbal fluency and executive functioning but equally impaired on language and episodic memory.

In conversation, people with Dementia with Lewy Bodies will present with reduced speech and word-finding difficulties, but no pragmatic difficulties (Rousseaux et al., 2010). The content of their hallucinations could also intrude into conversation and it may or may not be valuable to challenge these hallucinations during the conversation. However, one should monitor levels of distress carefully, and at times it may be more appropriate to distract people or reassure them in conversation (Alzheimer's' society website, 2012).

Parkinson's dementia

Parkinson's disease is caused by associated neuronal loss in the substantia nigra, which produces an inhibitory neurotransmitter – dopamine. It is a progressive neurodegenerative disease of older adults. The hallmark of this disease is the resting tremor, badykinesia, rigidity and postural instability. Dementia develops in 18–30% of people with Parkinson's disease, but between 30 and 40%, and perhaps up to 50%, of people with Parkinson's disease will nevertheless develop some executive difficulties. It is worth noting that people with Parkinson's disease demonstrate very early difficulties in some pragmatic skills, particularly processing emotional meanings and conveying them through facial expression and tone (Bourgeois & Hickey, 2009). Parkinson's disease dementia, however, will be characterized by loss of memory and reduced reasoning. Compared to people with Alzheimer's dementia, people with Parkinson's dementia present with more fluctuations and slower processing. They present with more executive difficulties but less language impairment.

Progressive Supranuclear Palsy (PSP)

Progressive Supranuclear Palsy is occasionally also known as Steele-Richardson-Olszewski syndrome and was first described as a separate condition from Parkinson's disease in 1964. The cause of PSP is unknown but its symptoms do overlap with Parkinson's disease (Alzheimer's society website, 2012). Recent research, however, indicates a link between environmental factors, such as tropical habitats, certain fruits and teas, and genetics (Zampieri & DiFabio, 2006). On neuropathological examination of patients who present with PSP, neurodegeneration, gliosis and abnormal collections of tau proteins can be observed, particularly in the basal ganglia, brain stem, pre-frontal cortex and cerebellum (Zampieri & DiFabio, 2006). PSP is distinguished from Parkinson's disease by the feature of vertical eye gaze paralysis, postural instability (falling backwards), significant speech and swallowing signs.

In PSP, executive impairments are the primary cognitive symptom and, combined with the frontal lobe dysfunction, mean that patients present as highly apathetic and disinhibited due to their poor self-monitoring (Bourgeois & Hickey, 2009). They also demonstrate very delayed processing and reduced memory (Zampieri & DiFabio, 2006; Alzheimer's society website, 2012). These changes can affect conversation just as much as the dysarthria that may be the more obvious problem when the patient is first referred to the speech and language therapist.

Korsakoff syndrome and Wernickes encephalopathy

Korsakoff syndrome is caused by a lack of thiamine (vitamin B12) to the brain. In the UK, it is most often caused by excessive alcohol consumption which results in either a very poor diet or damage to the lining of the stomach that then prevents absorption of the required nutrients. A lack of thiamine can also result in an episode of what is called Wernickes encephalopathy.

This is associated with Korsakoff syndrome and is often the precurser to the development of Korsakoff syndrome (Alzheimer's association website, 2012). Wernickes encephalopathy is sudden in onset, resulting in paralysis of muscles around the eyes, poor balance and drowsiness. If left untreated, Wernickes encephalopathy can result in permanent brain damage known as Korsakoff dementia. This damage occurs predominantly in the mid-brain structures. The hallmark of Korsakoff syndrome is memory loss but also involves other difficulties including learning new information and forming new memories, personality changes, limited insight and confabulations. It is these confabulations which in the past often resulted in people being described as suffering from Korsakoff psychosis.

People with Korsakoff syndrome present with cognitive communication difficulties in conversation characterized primarily by reduced memory of previous conversations. They will demonstrate little or no insight to this so that they are unable to continue a previous topic, and will perhaps assume incorrectly how much information or knowledge a listener may have on a subject. Their confabulations will intrude on conversation and they can become anxious and perseverative as a result. However, in comparison these patients will perform very well on formal assessment of communication.

Korsakoff syndrome can remain stable and not progress further if the individual ceases drinking, and adopts a healthier lifestyle. Some patients may even make some recovery from the condition, and it has been shown that around a quarter make a good recovery, whilst some recover a little and others will make no recovery (Alzheimer's association website, 2012).

HIV and AIDS dementia

HIV (Human Immunodeficiency Virus) and AIDS (Acquired Immunodeficiency Virus) are infections that weaken the immune system. This means the body finds it hard to fight off infection and illness. Cognitive changes can be caused by a number of different things, including cancers and other infections. It has, however, been found that the HIV virus does directly affect the brain, which may result in some cognitive changes such as delayed processing (Alzheimer's society website, 2012). A small number of patients may develop HIV and AIDS dementia. A diagnosis of HIV-associated neurocognitive disorders (HAND) is determined by the presence of difficulties in at least five areas of neurocognitive functioning known to be affected by the HIV infection, including executive functions, episodic memory, speed of processing, attention, memory, language, motor skills and sensoriperception (Woods, Moore, Weber & Grant, 2009). It is considered to have progressed to HIV-associated Dementia (HAD) when at least three of these areas have progressed to become moderate-to-severely impaired.

People with HIV don't generally present with any speech or language difficulties according to the majority of the literature. However, there is an increasing number of case studies which indicate otherwise. Indeed, Woods et al. (2009) cite a number of studies that describe an ataxic dysarthria in people with HIV. This is thought to include irregular rhythm and reduced vocal control of volume and perhaps a vocal tremor. Voice changes have also been described elsewhere in the literature (McCabe, Sheard & Code, 2006). This is mirrored in other clinical literature, which describes people with HIV as having slow and laboured speech (Bourgeois et al., 2009). It is important to remember that the cognitive deficits present in people with HIV-associated dementia will include reduced attention and concentration, reduced memory and speed of processing and loss of initiation. These will all impact upon conversation and social interactions. There is also some evidence that reduced processing – bradyphrenia, and perhaps impaired semantic memory – may affect verbal fluency, particularly verb generation (Woods et al., 2009).

HIV often targets the brain and the central nervous system because cells there express chemokine receptors that allow HIV entry into cells. Once HIV has crossed the blood–brain barrier it can cause synaptodendritic injury through its viral proteins and neuroinflammatory processes (Woods et al., 2009). HIV and AIDS dementia are caused by cerebral atrophy to the frontal, parietal and temporal regions with enlarged ventricles in the frontal and temporal regions. These patients present with enlarged multinucleated giant cells in the frontal and temporal regions and small inflammatory nodules in the white matter and sub-cortical nuclei (Bourgeois et al., 2009). This sub-cortical impairment in HIV and AIDS dementia (similar to that seen in Parkinson's or Huntington's dementia) results in slowed processing and impaired attention (McCabe et al., 2006). McCabe et al. (2006) hypothesize that sub-cortical impairments will also result in pragmatic communication impairments such as reduced prosody, fluency, difficulties with lexical selection, increased pauses, turn-taking difficulties and poor topic maintenance.

HIV and AIDS dementia can be improved and stabilized with the introduction of the right combination of anti-retroviral medications (Woods et al., 2009). It has also been reported that therapeutic rehabilitation such as physiotherapy, neuropsychology, occupational therapy and speech and language therapy can maximize these outcomes (Alzheimer's society website, 2012).

Table 2.2 Summary of dementia subtypes and the impact on communication.

*Cortical – symptoms patterns that result in aphasia, apraxia, agnosia, and amnesia. Sub-cortical – symptom patterns that result in bradyphrenia, mood disturbances and personality changes. These distinctions are no longer commonly used as diagnostic processes are becoming more sensitive and more specific diagnosis emerge where both cortical and sub-cortical structures are involved.

Predominantly cortical/sub-cortical*	Type of dementia	Characteristics of cognition and communication
Cortical	Alzheimer's (insidious decline)	Memory deficits, initially short term then more long term. Dysexecutive impairment WFD initially, then more significant global impairments (also likely personality and psychiatric changes)
Cortical and/or sub-cortical	Vascular (stepwise deterioration in function)	Focal communication difficulties may include speech, language and executive difficulties. (also risk of depression, anxiety and apathy)
Cortical	Frontotemporal dementia and primary progressive aphasias	FTD: progressive changes in behaviour PPA: progressive change in language and speech including semantic impairment (svPPA), dysfluency and agrammatism (navPPA), and phonological impairment (lvPPA) depending on the subtype
Cortical and sub-cortical	Lewy Body Dementia	Early attentional difficulties and hallucinations Reduced speech and word-finding difficulties Dysarthria will also impact on conversation
Sub-cortical	Parkinson's dementia	Primarily characterized by reduced memory, reduced reasoning and executive difficulties. NB: People with Parkinson's disease without dementia will also develop some pragmatic and executive difficulties. Dysarthria and dysphonia will also impact on conversation
Cortical and sub-cortical	Korsakoff syndrome	Memory difficulties are the hallmark, but confabulations and limited insight will all impact significantly on conversation
Sub-cortical	AIDS dementia	Reduced attention and concentration, reduced memory and speed of processing and loss of initiation. Language also worsens and patients can develop slow, laboured dysarthric and dysphonic speech
Sub-cortical	Progressive supranuclear palsy	Executive cognitive difficulties and frontal behaviours. Conversation is primarily characterized by apathy and disinhibition. Dysarthria and dysphonia will also impact on conversation.

Planning an assessment

The RCSLT UK position paper on dementia recommends that assessment of this client group should consider the following areas:

> "...evaluating a case history, pragmatics, discourse, use of referents, repetition of speech, paucity of speech, turn-taking, non-verbal skills, topic change/maintenance, confabulation, verbal fluency, sequencing, verbal reasoning, environmental impacts, family, language comprehension and reading."

This sounds much like the assessment we would undertake with any one of our patients who present with a stroke or brain injury, so many of the same assessment tools can apply. Be mindful, however, that many of the formal and standardized tools have not been specifically developed for people with dementia. Moreover, when you are planning assessment, this should always be guided by the patient's concern. Listen to what the patient is saying: "I am worried I keep forgetting names", or they report that they miss reading the paper as they can no longer "concentrate on it". These are therefore the most important areas for assessment. A good case history and evaluation of the communication environment, conducted prior to choosing an assessment, is invaluable at this stage (Tonkovich, 1999). What is the point in extensively assessing absolutely every domain of someone's communication when they really only wish to work on their word finding for work, or their ability to read their favourite paper? Endless assessment is not necessarily patient-centered nor worthwhile, whilst understanding your patient's needs and desires to support you in setting proper goals for therapy is vital.

Case history

Taking a proper case history is incredibly valuable in providing you with background information on the patient's current medical and social situation. This needs to be gathered from the patient's medical records but also verbally from the individual and/or from their family and carers. The patient's medical and social background needs to be considered alongside their clinical presentation in order to assist you in building a hypothesis about their difficulties. The patient's medical and social background will also influence their goals and management options.

Taking a complete social and medical history can be time consuming. Ideally, putting aside an entire session to talk with patients about their personal and social history is helpful, but not often realistic. However, these types of conversation can not only help you build rapport and a relationship with patients and their families, but also allow you to screen their communication before you choose an assessment. And indeed, formal assessment tasks may be intimidating and overwhelming for some individuals so gaining their confidence prior to carrying these out is very helpful.

Table 2.3 provides a few ideas on topics and questions you might find useful when collecting a social and medical history. It is not your responsibility to diagnose someone with dementia but it is valuable to understand what can influence someone's presentation. These are things a patient or their family members may mention to you and, if necessary, you can flag with appropriate medical teams such as neurologist, GP or geriatrician.

Generally, a diagnosis of dementia takes some time (even years) to assess by a specialist medical team, and can include blood testing, CT, MRI and even PET scanning. Neuropsychology and speech and language therapy assessment may also form part of this, particularly if the individual has been seen in a memory clinic or specialist centre. However, if you see a patient in your clinic, on the wards or at home and you seriously suspect they may have dementia it is vital you try to refer them on to the appropriate services. Unfortunately, some people may decline this. Other patients may already have a vague diagnosis that has 'appeared' at some point in their medical record. This can be much more tricky to deal with, yet warrants specialist assessment if the patient chooses. However, it is of course ultimately the patient's choice (if they have capacity) about how to pursue this.

Table 2.3 Ideas for taking a case history.

Medical history (Information can be gathered from medical records, conversation with patient, family or carers)

Do you have any other medical issues or problems we should be aware of? (*You may need to provide examples*)

Any other neurological issues or events? (*Big hint if they have Parkinson's disease or MS as this could be impacting on their thinking and they may not understand this is part of the disease process*)

Are you diabetic? (*Increased risk of stroke – multiple strokes can be linked with vascular dementia*)

(Continued overleaf)

Do you have arthritis or physical difficulties? (*Valuable to know how their lifestyle may be physically affected as well as cognitively*)

Any blood pressure issues? (*Again, increased risk of vascular dementia*)

Any old head injuries? (*Increased risk of dementias, particularly frontal variants*)

Any recent falls? (*Did they hit their head? What was the cause of the fall? Have they been well recently? This may highlight any new changes in physical as well as cognitive function*)

How's your mood (and mental state) been recently? (*Signs of depression can mimic cognitive decline – and may be treatable, or in conditions such as Parkinson's and Parkinson's plus syndromes can arise before other clinical signs are noticed*)

Any problems with thyroid function, or deficiency in vitamin B, etc? (*Any other metabolic or nutritional issues? A lack of some vitamins and changes in hormone function can mimic dementia symptoms. These symptoms are often reversible once the condition is appropriately treated*)

Any cancers? (*A patient who has had other cancers may be at increased risk of metastases which, when they arise in the brain, may cause significant cognitive impairment*)

Any recent infections (UTI, encephalitis, etc)? (*Infection can cause delirium which can be mistaken for cognitive changes, and is treatable*)

Any problems with oesophageal or bowel function? (*Unlikely to have a direct effect but again any type of infection can increase risk of delirium*)

Any recent operations? (*Some elderly people find anaesthesia has an increased impact on their cognition post-operatively*)

What medications are you currently taking? (*Some drug side effects and interactions can cause symptoms that mimic a dementia but, once adjusted, may be reversible*)

Any excessive alcohol consumption (or substance abuse) issues? (*People with long-term dependency have increased risk of cognitive decline and dementia*)

Have any of your close relatives had debilitating conditions; mother, father or siblings particularly? (*If a close family member has had the disease there may be an increased likelihood they will have it – although this is mainly only true if this is a first degree relative*)

Have you seen a speech and language therapist before? If so, what did you do with them?

Would you like me to explain what a speech and language therapist does? (*This can be a helpful part of an initial session, and help build trust and rapport*)

Social history

Where do you live and with whom?

Where were you born and where did you grow up?

Do you have a family? And where are they?

Does anyone help you out in day-to-day life? Who is this person? What do they do for you?

Who do you talk to or see regularly – do you have friends who you talk to?

What are your interests or your hobbies at present?

What were your interests and hobbies in the past (and why did you stop)?

What do you spend your time doing?

What is/was your occupation? What did this involve?

What was your education like? Where did you go to school/college/complete apprenticeship?

Did you do any more education or training after this?

Do you speak any other languages?

Communication history

What is the problem? What is worrying you?

When does this problem occur?

What happens? (*ask for specific examples*)

Has your communication changed over time? How long? Suddenly/gradually?

How is conversation – do people understand you?

Do you understand others?

How is your reading and writing?

What are your hobbies?

What do you do every day?

What do you do in the morning?

Do you go out in the day, if so who is there?

Do you talk to them or ask them anything?

What happens...why...?

What do you do to try to manage your communication difficulties in these situations?

Does it make a difference?

What do friends and family do to try to help you communicate?

Is this helpful?

What happens if they don't try to help?

How would you describe your personality and interaction style now? Is this different to previously?

What would you like to work on or improve in terms of communication?

What aspects of your life would you like to be better or different?

What would you like to work on in therapy?

What are your priorities for therapy?

Environmental evaluation (Information can be gathered from patient, family, nursing staff and from observation)

Is the environment sensitive to the person's communication needs – do people talk for him?

Are there 'restrictive rules' in place, e.g. don't talk to certain residents?

Are there qualified or willing communication partners around?

Does the person have a reason to talk?

Does the individual feel their contributions are meaningful?

Is there a lack of privacy?

Is there a lack of activity?

Is there anything that can cause sensory confusion and deprivation in the environment?

Is the person socially isolated?

Does the environment support the needs of the person's caregivers?

[Guided by Lubinski's (1995) list of factors comprising a communication impaired environment cited by Tonkovich, 1999]

Assessment

Once you have had this initial discussion you will be thinking about choosing your assessment approach. Part of this decision-making process will involve prioritizing what information you need to collect rather than planning what you wish to collect. Using multiple assessment tools to complete an in-depth analysis of all areas of expressive and receptive communication may provide you with a detailed understanding of their impairments, but is not always necessary or required (Tonkovich, 1999). Completing a less detailed communication assessment first, then choosing what you need to investigate in depth might be a good approach. The Comprehensive Aphasia Test, for example, was partly designed as a screen to guide you in deciding on further testing (Howard, Swinburn & Porter, 2009). However, when time is more pressing (either a limited number of sessions available or the person's ability and tolerance to engage is limited), you might be even more selective in your assessment choice: why assess reading at all if the individual doesn't have any interest in working on this skill and becomes tearful or frustrated when you try?

Yet don't forget the importance of formal assessment; language batteries provide a clinician with a summary of the individual's abilities and impairments, which together with the other information you collect allows you to begin hypothesizing about the nature of communication breakdown. It can allow you to decide on appropriate management strategies and monitor any changes (Howard et al., 2009).

Once you have identified the areas you are going to assess and you have an idea of the patient's approximate communication level from your informal assessment and observations during case history discussions you can select from a whole host of tools. Assessment tools vary widely in their focus, length and application so take care to choose an appropriate tool for your patient (American Speech-Language-Hearing Association, 2005; Shipley & McAfee, 2009). Table 2.4 provides a list of ideas of assessment tools you may find helpful. This is by no means exhaustive, but simply summarizes some of the more commonly available tools.

Table 2.4 List of assessment tools and ideas that may be useful.

Assessment*	Brief descriptions
Cognitive Linguistic Quick Test (CLQT: Helm-Estabrooks, 2001) (Standardized test for patients with dementia)	This tool is not specifically designed for assessing people with dementia and the norms are based on brain injury, stroke and Alzheimer's disease. However, it is a quick test examining orientation, attention, memory, naming, comprehension and executive difficulties. Recommended as a screening tool for speech and language therapists assessing communication in dementia by Shipley (2009).
Arizona Battery for Communication Disorders of Dementia (ABCD: Bayles & Tomoeda, 1993) (Standardized test for patients with dementia)	Specifically standardized on patients with dementia (Alzheimer's disease and Parkinson's disease without dementia). It is designed to assess a broad range of aspects of communication in dementia using a screen and then 14 subsets that focus on areas such as memory, verbal learning and visuo-spatial construction as well as expression and comprehension. The ABCD is frequently used in the literature with people with dementia (Jokel et al., 2009). It is also recommended for speech and language therapists working with people with dementia by Shipley (2009). However, it can be very long and may not identify functional needs (Bourgeois et al., 2009).
Comprehensive Aphasia Test (CAT; Swinburn, Porter, & Howard, 2004)	CAT includes sections on cognitive-linguistic skills, language skills and how the individual perceives their disability. This is standardized on patients with non-progressive aphasia (Howard, Swinburn & Porter, 2009). I, and many colleagues, have frequently used this with patients with dementia, particularly PPA, and found it very useful. It is moderately long but easily completed in stages.

(Continued overleaf)

Psycholinguistic Assessment of Language Processing in Aphasia (PALPA; Kay, Lesser, & Coltheart, 1992)	Aims to identify the precise point(s) of breakdown in language processing through examination of specific psycholinguistic functions. Can be used to refine your hypothesis of breakdown level (particularly with patients with PPA). This tool is used after screening communication using an alternative assessment, identifying areas that require further investigation and using different subsections of the PALPA to further investigate these areas.
Boston Naming Test (BNT, 3rd ed.; Kaplan, Goodglass, & Weintraub, 2000)	Designed to test naming with an hierarchy of prompting (semantic and phonological). Has been used in the research literature to assess naming in different types of dementia (Gorno-Tempini et al., 2008)
Boston Diagnostic Aphasia Examination – 3 (Goodglass, Kaplan, & Barresi, 2000)	An assessment tool that examines of all aspects of language, speech and includes reading and writing across more than 40 subsets. It is designed to be used with patients with non-progressive aphasia but has been used in the research literature with patients with dementia, particularly PPA (Jokel et al., 2009)). Unfortunately, it too is rather long for use with people with dementia (Bourgeois et al., 2009).
Western Aphasia Battery – Revised (WAB; Kertesz, 2006)	An assessment of language skills, again rather long for use with dementia patients. Commonly used with patients with non-progressive aphasia but has been used in the research literature with patients with dementia (Gorno-Tempini et al., 2008).
Pyramids and Palm Trees Test (Howard & Patterson, 1992)	Designed to clarify semantic knowledge without depending on spoken words, can be useful when refining an understanding of which variant of PPA someone may have such as svPPA. Has been used in the research literature with people with PPA (Giorno-Tempini et al., 2008).
Peabody Picture Vocabulary Test – 4th ed. (PPVT-4; Dunn & Dunn, 2007)	Designed to assess word comprehension, it has been used in the research literature to assess people with dementia (Jokel et al., 2009).

Burns Brief Inventory of Communication and Cognition (Burns Inventory; Burns, 1997)	Has three profiles of which the complex neuropathology inventory is specifically designed with dementia in mind.
Barnes Language Assessment (Bryan, Binder, Dann, Funnell, Ramsey, & Stevens, 2001)	Designed by the SIG Psychiatry of Old Age members (South of England), the Barnes Language Assessment was designed to profile language skills and difficulties in older adults with dementia.
Functional Linguistic Communication Inventory (FLCI; Bayles & Tomoeda, 1994) (Standardized test for patients with dementia)	Designed to be used with people with dementia but only standardized on people with Alzheimer's disease. Often more useful for people later in the disease process who cannot participate in formal assessment. Focuses on functional tasks, highlighting types of cues that can help, but may be too de-contextualized to provide true reflection of function (Bourgeois & Hickey, 2009).
Rivermead Behavioural Memory Test, 3rd ed. (Wilson, Greenfield, Clare, Baddeley, et al., 2008) (Standardized test for patients with dementia)	Focuses primarily on tasks that depend on memory. But, as with the FLCI, tasks may be too de-contextualised to reflect true performance.
CADL-2 Communicating Activities of Daily Living-2 (Holland, Frattali, & Fromm, 1999)	Originally designed as an assessment of the individual's abilities to communicate in functional communication situations, it has been shown to be useful working with acquired neurological conditions including stroke, brain injury and dementia. It is also recommended by Shipley & McAfee (2009) for speech and language therapists working with people with dementia. However, similar to the FLCI and Rivermead, tasks may be so out of context to not reflect true function.
The Functional Assessment of Communication Skills for Adults (ASHA FACS; Frattali, Holland, Thompson, Wohl, & Ferketic, 1995)	This was designed to assess everyday communication abilities in adults with communication difficulties. It includes rating scales of functional activities and asks you to rate these in four domains including social communication, communication of basic needs, reading, writing and numeracy as well as daily planning skills.

(Continued overleaf)

Discourse analysis/Conversation analysis (See discussion below)	Discourse analysis involves assessment of 'naturally occurring language'. This type of communication assessment is less formal. Some authors have published methods of analysis of discourse for people with different types of dementia (Arkin & Mahendra, 2001; Wong et al., 2009). However, models from aphasia rehabilitation may also apply to the dementia client group.
Conversation checklists	Pragmatics Profile (Dewart & Summers, 1996). Latrobe Communication Questionnaire (Douglas, O'Flaherty and Snow, 2000). Holden Communication Scale (Holden & Woods, 1995): checklists from the brain injury workbook or self-designed checklists can all be used with people with different types of dementia. The Holden Communication Scale is frequently used in the research literature to assess communication in people with dementia (Woods et al., 2012). The Pragmatics profile has also been used with some variants of dementia, including HIV/AIDS dementia (Woods, Moore, Weber, & Grant, 2009).
Communication in functional activities	Communication in activities of daily living may involve aspects of discourse analysis but is less structured and more patient centered. However, it is important to bear in mind that the clinician administering the task may bias interpretation and analysis of results in these types of assessment approaches (Bourgeois & Hickey, 2009).

*Including: Formal and standardized impairment-based assessment tools, formal and standardized functional assessment tools and more informal assessment tools.

NB: The tests that have been standardized for patients with dementia have been labelled as such. Many of the other tests may be standardized, but not with the dementia population.

Formal assessments

The American Speech-Language-Hearing Association advocates that assessment of people with dementia should examine "cognitive-communication strengths and weaknesses, including language comprehension and expression and integrity of working, declarative and non-declarative/procedural memory systems". Identifying both the strengths and weaknesses of the individual you are assessing allows you to judge their areas of need and their potential for different intervention approaches (American Speech-Language-Hearing Association, 2005; Bourgeois & Hickey, 2009). It also ensures you can provide appropriate advice to family members or carers about communication strategies to support conversation.

It is generally recommended that speech and language therapists choose assessment tools that are standardized or designed for the population they are working with to ensure results are sensitive and valid (American Speech-Language-Hearing Association, 2005).

Unfortunately, there are only a few test batteries that have been developed for speech and language therapists to use with patients with dementia. Murray and Clark (2005) attribute this to the fact that formal assessment tools for speech and language therapists working with dementia have only started to be published over the last 15 years. This also means that the majority of tools available are generally designed for people with Alzheimer's disease, this being the most common form of dementia (Murray & Clark, 2005). It is only very recently that tools such as the Northwestern Anagram Test (NAT) (Weintraub, Mesulam, Wieneke, Rademaker, et al., 2009) and the primary progressive aphasia Severity Scale (PASS) have been developed and are being used and validated as reliable measures for patients with primary progressive aphasia (Dickerson, 2011).

There are a number of formal assessment tools available on the market and they can have the great advantage of providing an overview of a patient's communication difficulties, support or clarify the communication features for diagnosis and are easily communicated to other professionals (Bourgeois & Hickey, 2009). Unfortunately, the perfect tools for your patient group are not always the tools available to you; indeed, you may need to clarify certain aspects of your assessment hypothesis using tools that are not specifically designed for this patient group.

It is important to be able to pick and choose the best assessment tool for your patient. To do this, it is also important to be able to weigh up the strengths and weaknesses of the tool you are using. Some tools will be biased to different client groups – especially if the tool has been standardized with a certain patient group – be that age, social and cultural group or disease type. For example, the Boston Naming Test will include items that are less familiar to many of your British patients, the ABCD is geared toward patients with

Alzheimer's and does not include a full range of language tasks, whilst the CADL-2 asks testees to consider communication situations in driving, using vending machines and other day-to-day tasks that may be irrelevant to some individuals. Equivalently, as the clinician you can inadvertently bias results when using less formal assessment tools, simply in the way you record an event. So weighing up the rationale for your assessment and the most appropriate test available to you may take some consideration.

It is not within the remit of this book, however, to review all the tools available on the market. Table 2.4 highlights a number of assessment tools often available in clinical settings. This list should help you reflect on which tools you have that might suit your patient. You may choose more than one assessment, or parts of different ones. It is also valuable to consider less formal assessment approaches including discourse analysis, conversation and functional communication. These approaches to assessment may well complement your formal assessment.

Informal assessment: Discourse, conversation and functional communication

Ehrlich (1994) defines discourse as "naturally occurring language that extends beyond the sentence level or across sentences". Discourse analysis aims to assess this 'naturally occurring language' where formal and standardized assessments fail. Indeed, research has shown that utterances observed on formal assessment differ from utterances produced in peer conversation (Beeke, Maxim, Best, & Cooper, 2011). The more functional approach to assessment offered by discourse analysis attempts to explore the complex and real changes in individual styles of communication that language or cognitive impairment may affect. Shadden (1995) distinguished between five different types of discourse:

1. *Narrative discourse*: Explanation of an event or a series of events, e.g. when responding to "Tell me about your daily routine" or "What are some things you do once in a while?"

2. *Procedural discourse*: Explanation of how a task is accomplished, such as a series of steps when responding to "Tell me how you would make a cup of tea."

3. *Expository discourse*: Less structured and when someone just talks on a topic, for example when responding to "So tell me what you know about dementia."

4. *Conversational discourse*: Engaging in communication with others, e.g. when discussing a values-laden topic such as, "What would you do if..." and following this up with more questions.

5. *Descriptive discourse*: Description of elements presented in a stimulus, e.g. when describing the cookie theft picture from the Boston Diagnostic Aphasia Examination (BDAE). This type of task has been shown to be particularly sensitive to linguistic deficits in Alzheimer's disease (Arkin & Mahendra, 2001).

A number of articles have examined the discourse deficits of people with dementia which until recently focused mainly on a very limited number of discourse tasks such as descriptive discourse and procedural discourse. Ehrlich (1994) has critiqued many of these as being focused predominantly on memory-laden tasks and lacking specificity as to the subjects' diagnosis. In fact, these have predominantly focused on people with Alzheimer's dementia or just a generic 'dementia'.

The following discussion provides a few ideas of how discourse can be rated in the clinical setting with people with dementia, and refers you to particular examples from the literature. However, this is only a snapshot of the types of approaches you might use in discourse analysis, and I would encourage you to explore this area further through reading articles, finding resources and in discussion with your colleagues.

Checklists and rating scales

Examining responses in discourse analysis can be complex, particularly in a clinical setting where it might be unreasonable to spend too much time transcribing responses. Instead, a clinician might choose to observe an interaction and qualitatively rate or measure content using a rating scale or checklist (Bourgeois & Hickey, 2009). Arkin and Mahendra (2001) suggest a method of analyzing responses by examining the number of positive versus negative utterances for responses made by patients with Alzheimer's disease. They base this on Audrey Holland's study of aphasic patients, and include positive utterances as on topic, relevant responses or a topic-related topic change with a return to the original topic at some point. Neutral utterances are described as unelaborated yes/no answers, empty or ambiguous answers, don't know statements, apologetic statements about their own communication, questions that are off topic, social statements or related topic changes with no return to the topic. Finally, negative utterances are described as incomplete ideas, statements with an unclear meaning, unrelated topic changes, word-finding difficulties within an utterance, confabulations, incorrect statements and perseverative statements. Arkin and Mahendra (2001) recommend this type of discourse analysis as a measure of treatment outcome and disease progression in dementia, but they also warn of the variability in performance as being not only dependent on the disease process but also personality.

Wong et al. (2009) also describe an assessment framework for discourse analysis for use with patients with Alzheimer's disease and semantic dementia. They describe a checklist that allows clinicians to develop a profile of a patient's communicative effectiveness. Wong et al. (2009) describe how a clinician can qualitatively rate performance from discourse tasks and carer feedback. This involves first identifying how a patient is able to 'codify ideas', i.e. are they spontaneously generated ideas that create conversational interaction or fixed over learned reactions and routine social exchanges such as recurrent stereotyped phrases. They then highlight that there are six general functions of communication: exchanges that have a creative function and generate stories; conversational exchanges that ask questions to gather information or share information; statements of how you feel or think; social exchange; and more regulatory exchanges to control behaviour of others, e.g. "Could you please…". The authors suggest that by identifying areas of communicative effectiveness and difficulty the clinician can plan treatment so intervention can focus on maintaining particular skills such as focusing on personal and interactional skills.

Conversation analysis

Conversation analysis can also focus on the interactions between two people. This can focus on the communication of both the patient and their conversational partner, and is perhaps one of the most useful approaches to discourse analysis for this client group given the large number of studies that support training of communication partners in all types of dementia (see Chapter 6). Most articles focus on checklists such as the communication skills checklist described by Bourgeois et al. (2004), which required the research assistant to observe an interaction between carers and patients with dementia and monitor the complexity of instructions given, strategies used and method of introduction. This is something that you may wish to borrow, or you can develop yourself as an informal tool. However, there are other tools available that are transferable from the stroke and brain injury population. One example of this is the Supporting Partners of People with Aphasia in Relationship and Conversation (SPPARC) approach (Lock, Wilkinson, & Bryan, 2008). This is a model of analysis that focuses on areas of conversation breakdown and repair, turn taking and topic maintenance. It requires the dyad to make a video recording of a typical conversation and encourages the patient and their partner to participate in the evaluation process. Although there is no formal research into the use of this with people with progressive language difficulties, as yet it is a concept that can be modified to suit the needs of those clients.

Functional conversation tasks

Functional conversational tasks are often designed by clinicians in the course of therapy planning and may include a specific activity the patient has reported as difficult. This type of informal discourse assessment is as valuable as the more formal testing. Often a patient will be assessed using a formal tool first (such as the CLQT or the CAT) and, following a detailed case history, the individual may highlight an area of concern: "I am having difficulties using the telephone", or "I am no longer able to do the shopping on my own". What follows may be considered by some to be intervention but it starts with informal assessment where the clinician will ask the individual to perform part of or the entire task, perhaps with support from the clinician, hereby identifying what is difficult. The clinician may perhaps use a checklist to guide this initial attempt. But with repetition and problem solving around these difficulties this evolves to become a therapeutic activity. The description of the pre- and post-therapy measures of discussions about a television programme described by Cartwright and Elliott (2009) as part of the 10 therapy sessions is a good example of such a method of assessment.

In summary

The past two decades have seen a dramatic shift in the way people with dementia are regarded, and changes in labels for these patients can clearly influence attitudes and actions of the people around them who shape their lives (Kitwood, 1995). Not only are progressive aphasias being more accurately diagnosed, but other types of dementia are also being increasingly recognized as dementias. Many of these are a consequence of the cognitive difficulties present in progressive diseases such as Parkinson's disease and AIDS, for example. It is important for clinicians to understand that each dementia variant will present differently depending on the cortical or sub-cortical structures affected.

These are all patients who may have been referred to a speech and language therapist with swallowing difficulties, or may have even been referred to them with specific communication needs. Patients may have multiple concerns that we need to address, including dysphagia, speech, language and cognitive communication difficulties. In fact, clients may find it incredibly difficult to separate the idea of speech and cognition or cognition and language when they describe difficulties in conversation. I remember the wife of one particular patient describing the difficulties her husband had in conversation. He had been diagnosed with PSP and he presented with both dysarthria, dysarthrophonia and cognitive communication difficulties. When we broke down these difficulties and explained that his articulatory difficulties were different to his difficulties in initiating conversational ideas she expressed such relief. She stated they seemed much more manageable this way. She also reported feeling a sense of validation – that there was more to his communication difficulties than the change in his speech. He had previously been such a joker, always the centre of conversation, a story-teller and dynamic guy. She felt his personality had changed completely, and couldn't work out why.

It is worth considering the therapeutic and educational benefits of the assessment process in itself at this point. I have frequently found that when family members observe the assessment they are able to use this information to gain a better understanding of the difficulties faced by their loved one. They have the opportunity to observe the individual communicating with another person, focusing on a very specific task, perhaps failing on some less complex tasks and succeeding on more difficult ones. This can allow people to gain some insight to their loved one's communication strengths and weaknesses. However, it is worth being prepared for family members who feel this assessment is not a true representation of their loved one's functions. This may be useful information – does this individual perform better in context? Or is this family member having difficulties adjusting and needs further education, counselling and support perhaps?

So as clinicians we should be somewhat prepared for the different types of impairments we might expect to observe in patients with different dementias, particularly in terms of cognition and communication. This knowledge complements assessment outcomes and is important to help you in supporting and educating patients and their families on communication strategies (Arkin & Mahendra, 2001) as well as preparing appropriate therapeutic interventions.

References

Alzheimer's society website (2012) Downloaded from http://www.alzheimers.org.uk/dementiamap and http://www.alzheimers.org.uk/site/scripts/news_article.php?newsID=1164

American Speech-Language-Hearing Association (2005) The roles of speech-language pathologists working with individuals with dementia-based communication disorders: Technical report. Available from www.asha.org/policy.

Arkin, S. & Mahendra, N. (2001) Discourse analysis of Alzheimer's patients before and after intervention methodology and outcomes. *Aphasiology* **15**, 533–569.

Bayles, K. A. and Tomoeda, C. K. (1993) *Arizona Battery for Communication Disorders of Dementia (ABCD)*. PRO-ED.

Bayles, K. A. & Tomoeda, C. K. (1994) *Functional Linguistic Communication Inventory (FLCI)*. PRO-ED.

Beeke, S., Maxim, J., Best, W., & Cooper, F. (2011) Redesigning therapy for agrammatism: Initial findings from the ongoing evaluation of a conversation-based intervention study. *Journal of Neurolinguistics* **24**, 222–236.

Bonner, M. F., Ash, S. & Grossman, M. (2010) The new classification of primary progressive aphasia into semantic, logopenic, or nonfluent/agrammatic variants. *Curr Neurol Neurosci Rep* **10**, 484–490.

Bourgeois, M. S. and Hickey, E. M. (2009) *Dementia: From Diagnosis to Management: A Functional Approach*. New York: Psychology Press.

Bourgeois, M. S., Dijkstra, K., Burgio, L. D. and Allen, R.S. (2004) Communication skills training for nursing aides of residents with dementia: The impact of measuring performance. *Clinical Gerentologist* **27** (1/2).

Braak, H., Alafuzoff, I., Arzberger, T., Kretschmar, H., & Tredici, K.D. (2006) Staging of Alzheimer disease associated with neurofibrillary pathology using brain sections and immunocytochemistry. *Acta Neuropathol* **112** (4), 389–404.

Brambati, S. M., Ogar, J., Neuhaus, B. L., and Gorno-Tempini, M. L. (2009) Reading disorders in Primary Progressive Aphasia: A behavioural and neuoimaging study. *Neuropsychologia* **47** (8–9), 1893–1900.

Bryan, K., Binder, J., Dann, C., Funnell, E., Ramsey, V., & Stevens, S. (2001) Development of a screening instrument for language in older people (Barnes Language Assessment). *Aging & Mental Health* **5**(4), 371–378.

Burns, M. (1997) *Burns' Brief Inventory of Communication and Cognition*. Pearson.

Cartwright, J. & Elliott, K. A. E. (2009) Promoting strategic television viewing in the context of progressive language impairment. *Aphasiology* **23**(2), 266–285.

Cotter, V. T. (2005) Alzheimer's disease: Issues and challenges in primary care. *Nursing Clinics of North America* **41** (1), 83–93.

Croot, K. (2009) Progressive language impairments: Definitions, diagnoses, and prognoses. *Aphasiology* **23**(2), 302–326.

Dewart, H. & Summers, S. (1996) Pragmatics profile of everyday communication skills in adults. Downloaded from: http://wwwedit.wmin.ac.uk/psychology/pp/

Dickerson, B. C. (2011) Quantitating severity and progression in Primary Progressive Aphasia. *J Mol Neuroschi.* **45**, 618–628.

Douglas, J. M., O'Flaherty, C. A. and Snow, P. C. (2000) Measuring perception of communicative ability: The development and evaluation of the La Trobe Communication Questionnaire. *Aphasiology* **14**(3), 251–268.

Dunn, L. M. & Dunn, D. M. (2007) *Peabody Picture Vocabulary Test*, 4th ed. (PPVT-4). Pearson.

Fletcher, P. (November, 2012) Speech and Language Therapy Psychiatry of Old Age Special Interest Group Study Day, November 2012, London.

Frattali, M. Holland, A. L., Thomson, C. K., Wohl, C., & Ferketic, M. (1995) *The Functional Assessment of Communication Skills for Adults* (ASHA FACS). American Speech-Language Hearing Association.

Goodglass, H., Kaplan, E., & Barressi, B. (2000) *Boston Diagnostic Aphasia Examination*, 3rd ed. (BDAE-3). Pearson.

Gorno-Tempini, M. L., Brambati, S. M., Ginex, V., Ogar, J., Dronkers, N. F., Marcone, A., Perani, D., Garibotto, V., Cappa, S. F., & Miller, B. L. (2008) The logopenic/phonological variant of primary progressive aphasia. *Neurology* **71**(16), 1227–1234.

Gorno-Tempini, M. L., Hillis, A. F., Weintraub, S., Kertesz, A., Mendez, M., Cappa, S. F., Ogar, J. M., Rohrer, J. D., Blacks, S., Boere, B. F., Manes, F., Dromkers, N. F., Vandenberghe, R., Rascovsky, K., Patterson, K., Miller, B. L., Knopman, D. S., Hodges, J. R., Mesulam, M. M., & Grossman, M. (2011) Classification of Primary Progressive Aphasia and its variants. *Neurology* **76**(11), 1006–1014.

Helm-Estabrooks, N. (2001) *Cognitive Linguistic Quick Test*. Pearson.

Hodges, J. R., Mitchell, J., Dawson, K., Spillantini, M. G., Xuereb, J. H., McMonagle, P., Nestor, P. J. & Patterson, K. (2010) Semantic dementia: Demography, familial factors and survival in a consecutive series of 100 cases. *Brain* **133** (1), 300–306.

Holden, U. P. &Woods, R. T. (1995) *Positive Approaches to Dementia Care*, 3rd ed. Edinburgh: Churchill Livingston.

Holland, A.L., Frattali, D., & Fromm, C. M. (1999) *Communication Activities of Daily Living*, 2nd ed. CADL-2. PRO-ED.

Howard, D. & Patterson, K. (1992) *Pyramids and Palm Trees Test*. Pearson.

Howard, D., Swinburn, K., & Porter, G. (2009) Putting the CAT out: What the Comprehensive Aphasia test has to offer. *Aphasiology* **24**(1), 56–74.

Huber, A., Stuchbury, G., Burkle, A., Burnell, J., & Munch, G. (2006) Neuroprotective therapies for Alzheimer's disease. *Current Pharmacological Design* **12**, 705-717.

Jokel, R. Cupit, J., Rochon, E., & Leonard, C. (2009) Relearning lost vocabulary in nonfluent progressive aphasia with MossTalk Words®. *Aphasiology* **23**(2), 175-191.

Kaplan, E., Goodglass, H., & Weintraub, S. (2000) *Boston Naming Test*, 3rd ed. Lippincott Williams and Wilkins.

Kay, J., Lesser, R., & Coltheart, M. (1992) *Psycholinguistic Assessment of Language Processing in Aphasia*. Hove: Psychology Press.

Kertesz, A. (2006) *Western Aphasia Battery – Revised (WAB)*. Pearson.

Kertesz, A., Jesso, S., Harciarek, M., Blaire, M., & McMonagle, P. (2010) What is semantic dementia? A cohort study of diagnostic features and clinician boundaries. *Arch Neurol.* **67**, 483-489.

Kitwood, T. (1995) Studies in person centered care: Building up the mosaic of good practice. *Journal of Dementia Care* **3**(5), 12-13.

Lock, S., Wilkinson, R., & Bryan, K. (2008) *Supporting Partners of People with Aphasia in Relationships and Conversation*. Milton Keynes: Speechmark.

McCabe, P., Sheard, C., & Code, C. (2006) Pragmatic skills in people with HIV/AIDS. *Disability and Rehabilitation* **29**(16), 1251-1260.

McKhann, G. M., Albert, M. S., Grossman, M., Miller, B., Dickson, D. & Trojanowski, J. Q. (2001) Clinical and pathological diagnosis of frontotemporal dementia. Report of the Work Group on Frontotemporal Dementia and Pick's Disease. *Arch Neurology* **58** (11), 1803-1809.

Mesulam, M. (2001) Primary progressive aphasia. *Annals of Neurology* **49** (4), 425-432.

Murray, L. & Clark, H. M. (2005) *Neurogenic Disorders of Language*. New York: Singular Publishing.

National Collaborating Centre for Mental Health commissioned by the Social Care Institute for Excellence National Institute for Health and Clinical Excellence (revised 2011) THE NICE -SCIE GUIDELINE ON SUPPORTING PEOPLE WITH DEMENTIA AND THEIR CARERS IN HEALTH AND SOCIAL CARE National Clinical Practice Guideline Number 42 published by The British Psychological Society and Gaskell. Downloaded from: http://www.nice.org.uk/nicemedia/live/10998/30320/30320.pdf

Neary, D., Snowden, J. S., Gustafson, L., Passant, V., Stuss, D., Black, S., Freedman, M., Kertesz, A., Robert, P. H., Albert, M., Boone, K., Miller, B. L., Cummings, J. & Benson, D. F. (1998) Frontotemporal lobar degeneration. A consensus on clinical diagnostic criteria. *Neurology* **51** (6), 1546-1554.

Neef, D. & Walling, A. D. (2006) Dementia with Lewy Bodies: An emerging disease. *American Family Physician* **1:73** (7), 1223-1229.

Papp, K. V., Walsh, S. J., & Snyder, P. J. (2009) Immediate and delayed effects of cognitive interventions in healthy elderly: A review of current literature and future directions. *Alzheimer's Dementia* **5**(1), 50–60.

Rousseaux, M., Seve, A, Vallet, M., Pasquir, F., & Mackowiak-Cordoliani, M. A. (2010) An analysis of communication in conversation in patients with dementia. *Neuropsychologia* **48**, 3884–3890.

Royal College of Speech and Language Therapists (2005) Speech and language therapy provision for people with dementia. RCSLT Position Paper. London: RCSLT. Downloaded from: www.rcslt.org/resources/publications

Salmon, E., Perani, D., Collette, F., Feyers, D., Kalbe, E., Holthoff, V., Sorbi, S., & Herholz, K. (2007) A comparison of unawareness in frontotemporal dementia and Alzheimer's disease. *BMJ* **79**, 176–179.

Shadden, B. B. (1995) The use of discourse analysis and procedures for communication programming in long-term care facilities. *Topics in Language Disorders* **15**, 75–86.

Shipley, K. G. & McAfee, J. G. (2009) *Assessment in Speech and Language Pathology: A Resource Manual*, 4th ed. Cengage Learning, Delmar, USA.

Spector, A. & Orrell, M. (2010) Using a psychosocial model of dementia as a tool to guide clinical practice. *Int Psychogeriatric* **22**(6), 957–965.

Swinburn, K., Porter, G. & Howard, D. (2004) *Comprehensive Aphasia Test (CAT)*. Hove: Psychology Press.

Taylor, C., Kingma, R. M., Croot, K., & Nickels, L. (2009) Speech pathology services for primary progressive aphasia: Exploring and emerging area of practice. *Aphasiology* **23**(2), 161–174.

Threats, T. World Health Organisation's International Classification of Function, Disability and Health: A framework for clinical and research outcomes. In: L. A. C. Golder & C. M. Frattali (2012) *Outcomes in Speech Language Pathology*, 2nd ed. New York: Thieme.

Tonkovich, J. D. (1999) Managing the long-term communication and memory consequences of dementia. *In Neurophysiology and Neurogenic Speech and Language Newsletter* **9**(5), 9–14.

Weintraub, S., Mesulam, M. M., Wieneke, C., Rademaker, A., Rogalski, E. J., & Thomson, C. K. (2009) The northwestern anagram test: Measuring sentence production in primary progressive aphasia. *Am. J. Alzheimer's Dis. Other Dementia* **24**, 408–416.

Wilson, B. A., Greenfield, E., Clare, L., Baddeley, A., Cockburn, J., Watson, P., Tate, R., Sopena, S., & Nannery, R. (2008) *Rivermead Behavioural Memory Test*, 3rd ed. London: Pearson.

Wong, S. B., Anand, R., Chapman, S. B., Rackley, A., & Zientz, J. (2009) When nouns and verbs degrade: Facilitating communication in semantic dementia. *Aphasiology* **23**(2), 286–301.

Woods, B., Aguirre, E., Spector, A. E., & Orrell, M. (2012) Cognitive stimulation to improve cognitive functioning in people with dementia. *Cochrane Database of Systematic Reviews 1.2*. The Cochrane Collaboration. Chichester: John Wiley & Sons.

Woods, S., Moore, D., Weber, E., & Grant, I. (2009) Cognitive neuropsychology of HIV-associated neurocognitive disorders. *Neuropsychol. Rev* **19**,152–168.

Zampieri, C. & DiFabio, R. P. (2006) Progressive supranuclear palsy: Disease profile and rehabilitation strategies. *Physical Therapy* **86**, 870–880.

3 Treatment planning and goal setting

Introduction

> "Speaking generally, there is nothing original about the concept of goal setting. Everyone knows that you have to set goals in order to accomplish anything in life. Goal-directedness is, after all, the distinctive feature of rational human activity" Locke, Cartledge, & Koeppel (1968)

In therapy, goal setting is the process of identifying an area of need and, together with the client, deciding what it is that therapy will aim to achieve in this area. Even though the individual with dementia may be living with a progressive deteriorating disease it remains important to set clear goals for therapy. Having said that, how do we as clinicians establish what the areas of need are, and how do we aim to treat them with this client group when their condition does continue to deteriorate?

Having a conversation about goal setting with a patient and their family members is never straightforward. There are many published and formalized models of goal setting that can support our therapy, some of which may be required of us in order to demonstrate our outcomes (in the current economic climate) at work. This chapter emphasizes the specific factors you may need to consider when goal setting and planning therapy with the progressive patient group, particularly those patients with communication difficulties. It suggests certain approaches to goal setting, with examples of the types of questions that can facilitate this phase of your therapy planning with your patient. These suggestions are by no means the only way to work on goal setting but aim to lay a foundation.

Thinking about goal setting with patients living with communication difficulties

Some clinicians assume that it is too complex or too difficult to set goals for patients with progressive communication difficulties such as those present in dementia. However, the Royal College of Speech and Language Therapy (RCSLT, 2005) recommends that speech and language therapy services providing care to patients with dementia should endeavour to "ensure the philosophy and goals of intervention are shared and consistent" across the team they are working with. The RCSLT provides examples of where it can be vital to set such goals:

> "In certain environments such as nursing facilities and inpatient wards it is important to set collaborative goals related to self care and interactions with staff."

Without proper advice on how to communicate with a patient, completing – let alone improving – areas that are difficult in basic personal care or nursing care tasks can be unnecessarily traumatic for both parties involved. Family at home may need a similar type of support. There will also be times when you will be asked to work directly with individual patients on improving their language and communication skills. It will be as important to set goals when working directly with patients as when you are working with the people around them.

As therapists working in rehabilitation will know, goal setting has been described and discussed extensively in the literature and it is not within our remit to provide a review of all of this information. The process of setting Specific Measurable Attainable Relevant Timely goals (SMART goals) is similar across different client groups. There are, however, some considerations specific to the dementia population that might influence this process. These are factors that may guide your planning and support the rationale for your goals. The following sections focus on some of the main themes from the literature around goal setting as well as some issues that will be more relevant to the dementia client group.

Relevant 'patient centered' goal setting

An issue that a clinician may consider relevant might not be so relevant for a patient. This can impact on the patient's motivation to engage in therapy and work on this goal. In general, it is important that a goal be of value to the patient, otherwise they may become despondent and disengaged from therapy. Thus, when goal setting with a patient with progressive language or communication impairment it is particularly valuable to consider what is really useful to that individual. For example, if you are considering working on naming skills then consider exactly what you are really aiming to achieve. Is the desired outcome that a patient be able to name objects or be able to continue using said objects? From a functional perspective there may be just as much of a need to know the use and function of this object as the name. Some authors suggest therapy in progressive language disorders should actually focus more on understanding functional attributes of objects as this could have a direct impact on maintaining the individual's independence in daily living for longer (Bier, Macoir, Gagnon, Van der Linden, et al., 2009).

In order to reflect the desired outcome, a goal should therefore articulate what you are aiming to achieve rather than just the method you will use to do this. This is a common mistake that clinicians make – documenting the therapy task such as 'completing daily naming exercises', rather than the end result: 'to be able to request the correct tool from my colleagues at work'.

Goals should also identify the desired outcome: what I will accomplish, not what I am going to avoid. By describing what will be accomplished the patient and their clinician can actually specifically define the outcome. This can, in turn, guide the measurement of the goal outcome. For example rather than 'I won't depend on my wife to talk so much' one might state, 'I will be able to order my own meal in a restaurant every time we go out for lunch next month'. This is a goal which will be clearly understood by a patient and their family, and can be measured by stating, for example, 'I ordered my own meal three of the four times we dined out last month'.

Achievable goal setting

Goals must also be achievable, as well as relevant. Yet they should not be too easy either. Guthrie and Harvey (1994) suggest that setting specific but challenging goals is the best way of motivating people at work. They also suggest that aiming high enhances self-esteem and increases effort and outcomes. The individual is invested and feels some ownership and responsibility for the goal. But some authors warn of having expectations that are too high with patients with progressive communication difficulties. Evidence shows that therapy tasks can improve and maintain word recall over time for patients with progressive language impairment. However, as the disease progresses these words will be lost even with maintenance exercises (Heredia, Sage, Sage, & Berthier, 2009). Unrealistic expectations can lead to communication breakdown and stress for all parties: patient, carers and clinician. If the SLT is able to provide intervention at specific stages of the progression of the disease they can thereby support and assist carers to develop more realistic expectations of maintaining skills for as long as possible and (hopefully) appropriate coping mechanisms for when things do continue to deteriorate (Barnes, 2003).

However, other authors such as Guthrie and Harvey (1994) advise the opposite. They suggest that unrealistically high goals resulting from denial may be an important protective response and should not necessarily be immediately confronted. They suggest that personal goals are linked with hope and optimism. If we deny a person their hope we may see very little motivation to make any change. Consequently, any expected progress may not happen at all. This may be particularly pertinent for patients with progressive communication difficulties.

When working with patients with progressive communication difficulties we need to revise our expectations of what patients will achieve in therapy. Papp, Walsh and Snyder (2009) highlight that, whilst we could expect non-progressive patients to achieve high levels of accuracy within sessions, we might need to reduce our expectations for patients with progressive diseases. That is, where patients with non-progressive conditions might achieve 95% accuracy on therapy targets before moving on, patients with progressive conditions might achieve only 75%. It might also be helpful to reconsider other factors such as timescales. Breaking goals into smaller sections that can be achieved within a reasonable amount of time initially may be helpful (Shut & Stam, 1994). This can meet both needs: patients are able to aim high and preserve their hope and optimism but continue to achieve the shorter-term goals, thus maintaining a sense of achievement and therefore motivation.

Croot et al. (2009) remind us, however, that there are a host of different factors that could affect motivation for this patient group, such as grief, insight, personality changes and previous personality factors. The emotional and psychological impact of progressive diseases can have a significant effect on therapy intervention over time. It seems that, as the disease progresses, ongoing therapy could become less of a priority. This is often a result of increased distress in response to therapy tasks that continually remind the patient of the disease he is living with. There are numerous examples of this in the literature. Graham, Pratt and Hodges (1998) describe how their case study (DM) initially worked to bolster his motivation by showing how he could actively be involved in improving his naming, i.e. if he participated in practice he could actually improve his word naming. However, the perpetual homework had the opposite effect over time, and resulted in periods of depression and frustration where he was painstakingly aware that he would lose words regardless of the amount of practice he did. DM became increasingly obsessed with adding words to his lists to practise. Not only did this impact on his mood but it also had a negative effect on his family.

Finally, simple physiological factors such as fatigue may also impact on therapy in this population. If a patient becomes quickly fatigued after 20 to 30 minutes then therapy needs to reflect this need, ensuring tasks take no longer than 20 to 30 minutes. This may, for example, restrict the number of words you target on a naming or comprehension task, or may influence the recommendations you give a family member. When setting goals with the patient or family these motivation and psychological factors need to be thoroughly considered.

Measurable goal setting

Goals can capture meaningful information such as the functional change on completing specific tasks, e.g. reading a paper, or increased confidence in a task (Kindell & Griffiths, 2006). If a patient is not achieving their goals this may indicate the goals were set too high, were unrealistic or that therapy is just not currently useful. This method allows you to evaluate what has changed for an individual. We must not forget that outcomes can also allow commissioners to monitor spending and compare facilities, so it is important to reflect on what has changed as a result of intervention.

The main premise behind goal setting is that some kind of positive change will occur to achieve the identified outcome. And many of the tools available that support the goal setting process, such as the Goal Attainment Scaling system for example, ask for a rating of where the patient is before and after using a therapy. Unfortunately, it can be significantly more difficult to quantify and reflect a positive change on such a rating scale for a patient living with progressive communication difficulties. Therapy may result in improvements but, similarly, a period of stability or slowing in deterioration could reflect the positive influence of therapy.

As therapy may result in slowing of deterioration, rather than noticeable improvement, it is vital that the person with progressive communication difficulties and their communication partners (be it family, friends, carers and staff) understand this possibility (Croot et al., 2009). Similarly, they should understand that therapy will not reverse progression either. Jokel, Cupit, Rochon and Leonard (2009) emphasize that research evidence in the area of naming therapy for progressive language impairments has shown proven maintenance of residual skills. So when you are developing a treatment plan around this type of therapy intervention, you can use this information to guide you in the language you use in goal setting.

Patients may also need to be told that the effects of therapy are unlikely to generalize to words, phrases and situations other than those targeted by the task at hand. A therapy that focuses on specific vocabulary or phrases is unlikely to generalize to other items. In comparison, an approach that targets more general rules of communication, such as cognitive communication strategies or syntactic rules, may be more likely to be transferred to other situations (Croot et al., 2009). However, the likelihood of carryover and generalization when working on therapy tasks, particularly impairment-based therapies, is limited. Even the literature for non-progressive language and communication difficulties demonstrates little or no generalization to untreated words (Croot et al., 2009). Consequently, goals also need to reflect the specific task being addressed in therapy.

Setting the actual goal with your patients

When should you start this conversation?

You will find differing literature, with some authors suggesting that goals can or should be set before any assessment takes place whilst others suggest otherwise. Whatever you decide will probably depend on how you work and what your patients prefer. With some you need the time in assessment to build rapport and gain a better understanding of how the person communicates to support that discussion, whilst other people will come to you with a clear idea of exactly what they want.

Treatment planning should be a collaborative process. Patients arrive at therapy with certain expectations and may demand or request what they feel they need from you, be it specific advice or your opinion on everything. I have experienced patients requesting intensive impairment-based programmes or advice on a therapy strategy they have already set up for themselves. It is quite common to receive these types of requests in clinical practice (Croot et al., 2009). And these types of requests are worth considering. The more a patient feels they have contributed to the planning of therapy the more 'buy in' there is likely to be. Moreover, there is a higher likelihood of patients actually carrying over therapy tasks to independent practice at home. Other patients may depend more on your advice as an 'expert'. They may expect and rely on you to decide on goals for them. Whilst they think they are leaving it up to the therapist, these patients will likely also benefit from being guided through a discussion around their ideas for goal setting.

Yet you may find that discussing goals is not such an easy thing to do. The more you practise the easier it will get. However, you will likely always find that there are some patients who take some time to tell you what their goal really is, only after they feel they can trust you, or they have had time to formulate their goal themselves.

Where to start? Identifying areas of need with your patient

Most goal-setting philosophies will encourage you to sit with the individual (and relevant family members or carers) to identify their priorities or aspirations for the future. Perhaps one of the most difficult practical aspects of this process is using the right vocabulary. Many patients will be familiar with what a 'goal' is whilst others may struggle with the concept. Some of the goal-setting tools available on the market can guide you down this path (Goal Attainment Scaling, Care Aims or Patient Reported Outcome Measures are described in more detail in Chapter 8). The Goal Attainment Scaling tool, for example, offers a useful worksheet to fill in as you are setting goals with a patient. Some tools will have standard questions to assist with this conversation, but nevertheless it can be tricky to apply these principles to patients with progressive communication difficulties.

As symptoms and disability increase for individuals with neurodegenerative disease, the more they become segregated and isolated from opportunities for cognitive stimulation within their community. This can be because they no longer hold their driver's licence or they have difficulty using public transport. They may experience embarrassment and loss of confidence in socialising with friends. This results ultimately in a loss of independence. People with aphasia report social isolation, loneliness, loss of autonomy, restricted activities, role changes and stigmatization (Cherney, Halper, Holland, & Cole, 2008). This loss in independence can hasten the rate of clinical decline as there are fewer opportunities to develop compensatory strategies and stimulate alternative synaptic networks. In order to provide ongoing opportunities for communication we need to identify what situations are motivating and appropriate for our patients (Cartwright & Elliott, 2009).

A starting point for a goal-setting conversation with patients with progressive diseases can be around identifying areas of need. What is particularly difficult? What has changed? What has improved? However, for many patients even this may be tricky to describe. Situations may have changed so much, and over such a long period, that it can be difficult to prioritize any area. Insight and expectations will also influence this conversation so striking a balance between what is valuable, what is realistic and what can result in a positive outcome can be tricky.

Most areas of concern that patients will identify will likely be very functional: "I want to be able to remember words better so I can talk to my friends at the pub", or "I want to be able to read letters", or "I want to be able to talk more quickly on the phone". Most daily communication activities can be addressed in speech and language therapy. Even activities such as watching television can become opportunities for therapy. Cartwright and Elliott (2009) describe a pilot for communication therapy that enhances the television watching experience.

Authors do highlight that, even if a patient is unable to participate in the goal setting discussion, it is legitimate to carry on the same discussion with their carers or relatives. They suggest that, as long as individuals are able to understand the tasks required, then they are likely to be suitable candidates for many therapies including impairment-based language therapy (Croot, 2009). Table 3.1 provides some ideas for appropriate questions to start discussing areas of need for goal setting.

Table 3.1 Ideas for questions to start discussing areas of need for goal setting.

Previous history	Current history	Future plans
Occupation What did you do for a living? Did you have to read/talk/write/use a computer a lot at work? *Living arrangements* What were your responsibilities around the home previously (e.g. doing the bills or the banking)? *Family/friends* What were you like previously (chatty/joker/listener, etc?) Did you previously spend a lot of time socializing? *Hobbies* What interests did you have previously? Has this changed? *Routine* Has anything changed in your daily routine? *Achievements/stories* Is there anything in your past that you were particularly proud of achieving? Or was there anything particularly important that you like to tell people about?	*Daily routine* What do you do each morning/afternoon/evening? Where do you buy your paper? How do you plan your shopping/meals? *Leisure activities* Do you have any particular hobbies or interests? What programmes do you watch on TV? What paper do you read? Who do you speak to on the phone? Who answers the phone/makes calls? Who do you socialize with and where? Do you speak to your family regularly? *People involved in care* Who do you live with? Who does your shopping/cleaning? What do you talk about? *Mood* How do you feel about your communication? *Impairment* What is the main problem with your communication? How is your speaking? How is your reading? How is your writing? How do you manage in understanding others: one-to-one or in groups?	*Family/friends* Who will you be seeing and chatting with in the near future and when? *Aspiration/dreams* What plans do you have for the near future? What would you like to achieve in the future?

Developing a goal

Once you have identified some areas that you have agreed are areas of difficulty you can consider how they can be addressed. From this, you may agree on the finer details of the goal itself. This could require guidance and coaxing and again may depend on the model of communication you are using. Sometimes, this can take the form of probing questions to help the patient to describe exactly what they may wish to improve or achieve. This process can feel as though you are providing a type of counselling, which indeed you may be for some individuals. Simple strategies such as active listening; using paraphrasing, summarizing and giving the patient an opportunity to talk are all skills that will assist in this process (Reid, 2012). However, there are other approaches which can enable you to become more skilled in this process. Other intervention approaches such as motivational interviewing, cognitive behavioural psychology and solution-focused therapy have all influenced the way I approach goal setting with my patients.

Having a few questions up your sleeve can be helpful:

- What do you wish to achieve in this area?
- How do you wish to change this?
- By when?
- What do you think speech and language therapy can do to help this?
- We have identified writing as a concern – what kind of things would you like to write?
- What words do you think it would be most useful to work on?
- So you often forget names. Would you like to be able to get people's names right independently in conversation at morning tea?

Once an agreement has been reached regarding what may be changed the process of forming an agreement about the goal itself can commence. More specific approaches such as SMART goal-setting techniques can provide a framework to the specific wording for the goal. SMART goal setting requires you to make goals Specific, Measurable, Attainable, Realistic and Timely. Having a repertoire of SMART-type goals that have been useful for other patients can provide you with a helpful list from which to seek ideas with future patients. Table 3.2 provides a list of goals that could be applicable to patients with progressive communication difficulties.

Table 3.2 Example goals.

Area of difficulty	Potential goals
Mealtimes at home with the family going out in public preparing meals making meal choices	To be able to request the salt/pepper at family meal times. To be able to order my own meal in a restaurant every time we go out for lunch next month. To be able to follow a basic recipe to prepare myself meals at home. To be able to express my preference for what meal I would like when my wife/husband asks.
Shopping talking to strangers shopping lists and packets	To be able to order and purchase the tools and materials I need from the hardware shop. To write my own shopping list so I can do my weekly shopping.
TV understanding and keeping up discussing programmes	To be able to understand the gist of a TV programme I am watching with my wife. To be able to discuss the television programs we watch with my wife.
Socializing with family with friends with staff and carers with strangers at clubs/hobbies	To remember the names of my family. To be able to talk to my grandchildren and ask them questions about their lives. For my family/partner to be confident and comfortable in talking with me. To remember the names of people at the morning coffee group, using a communication-memory book. To be able to tell a story with my wife's help, when we are out with friends. To be more confident in having a conversation with people I know. To be able to tell new people I meet why my communication is difficult. To be able to use my communication book to tell a story about what has happened in my life. To be able to remember suburbs and road names in areas in which I travel around.

(Continued overleaf)

Work	To be able to ask for and answer requests for tools at work.
	To be able to order and purchase the tools and materials I need from the hardware shop.
Telephone use with familiar people; with strangers; answering the phone; making a call; taking a message	To be able to plan and make a telephone call to a family member.
	To be able to take a message for my husband/wife when someone calls for them.
Reading the paper	To be able to read the newspaper headline every day.
Writing notes; lists; letters	To be able to take a message when someone calls.
	To be able to hand-write a letter to my sister.
	To write my own shopping list so I can do my weekly shopping.

Using goals to plan therapy

Whatever goals have been agreed upon, therapy planning must also be guided by the results and analysis of your assessment. An appropriate assessment tool can identify the individual's areas or strength and difficulties. This can in turn allow you to develop the most appropriate therapy programme to achieve the desired goal, for example, by using a psycho-linguistic assessment to clarify the cause of a naming difficulty. From this, the clinician is able to form a hypotheses such as: "This particular individual's naming difficulties are a result of a breakdown in semantic knowledge" (Croot et al., 2009). Then a useful therapy task might be to target semantic features of objects. This type of task can then be linked to the patient's priority. For example, the patient who wishes to continue their favourite leisure activity (bowling) for as long as possible, may benefit from working on specific object words and concepts he needs for this task.

On the odd occasion we do come across patients who state that they simply want to be able to name pictures and read single words. We must be able to identify what exactly these clients need these skills for. We cannot support someone in their wish to drive without knowing if it's going to be by bicycle, car, van or motorbike.

In fact, by being highly patient centered you will be more likely to identify highly functional therapy targets that are relevant and meaningful to the person's everyday life. Croot et al. (2009) cites a study by Snowden and Griffiths (2002) which indicated that a patient they worked with was more likely to make gains when learning was linked to personally meaningful environments and experiences. Basically, doing work in a person's own home and using their own belongings, working on meaningful and useful tasks is more likely to support maintenance of knowledge. This may be attributed to the idea that working on information associated with existing retained knowledge is more likely to be successful (Croot et al., 2009). This means therapy will not only be targeting retrieval, but also strengthening already stored skills or information. Croot et al. (2009) hypothesized that these links increase the likelihood of carryover to spontaneous speech and felt it was this repeated practice through spontaneous speech that in turn acted most effectively to maintain skills.

Case study: Ms A

Ms A was referred to speech and language therapy with a diagnosis of Primary Progressive Aphasia of the semantic variant. She was also diagnosed with depression. Her family reported she had previously been an extremely gregarious, sociable and determined woman who escaped poverty and an abusive father to come and live in a Western country with her husband. This determined nature was also reflected in how she encouraged each of her children to achieve academically and her motivation to also return to school to study English. However, over the last six years they described a progressive deterioration in her communication and her confidence.

At her first session, Ms A presented as a very quiet, shy woman, who whispered when she spoke and frequently looked to her daughter to communicate for her. Discussion around goal setting took place over two sessions as she slowly established confidence in her relationship with the therapist. Conversation highlighted:

- **Areas of need/concern**

    Feeling lonely and isolated

    Lack of understanding of what was happening to her communication

    Often crying and distressed by thoughts of her past but unable to talk about them

Feelings of boredom

Difficulties initiating activities or household chores, but able to complete routine tasks once prompted

Dependent on family for most aspects of daily tasks

Grief and loss feelings experienced by her family

Family felt unsure and anxious about how to talk with her

Her grandchildren would visit but she didn't know what to say to them and would often forget their names.

- **Areas of need that we agreed to work on**

  Families and patients understanding of the changes in communication

  Talking to her family and grandchildren

  Talking about the past

  Families' confidence in communicating with her.

- **What would be better/what needed to be changed**

  For Ms A and her family to understand the causes of changes in communication and be able to prepared for the future

  For the family to know what strategies to use in communicating with their mother/wife/grandmother

  For Ms A to remember her grandchildren's names

  For Ms A to be able to talk about the past.

- **Define the wording of your goal**

  ➔ For patient and family to demonstrate an understanding of progressive aphasia and how this impacts on their mother's or wife's communication in a conversation with the speech and language therapist

  ➔ For family members to feel more confident (as per self-rating) about how to have a conversation with their mother/wife

> → For Ms A to be able to call her grandchildren and children by their appropriate names most of the time in conversation at home (as per self-report most of the time means more than 50%)
> → For Ms A to be able to have a conversation with her family in which she can talk about events from her past.
>
> - **Discuss how you might achieve this**
>
>   An education session with the family following the assessment period
>
>   Training session with husband and daughter to provide an opportunity to practise conversation with Ms A
>
>   Naming therapy programme using photos of grandchildren (including home assignments)
>
>   Development of personal communication book (including home visit and home practice sessions).
>
> - **Agree on how long it might take**
>
>   8 weeks of therapy with one session per week.
>
> - **Commence therapy**
>
>   Date set to commence therapy and date set to review progress.

In summary

Goal setting and treatment planning with patients with progressive communication difficulties follows the same pattern as goal setting with any other patient group. And, as with any other case, deciding what goals to work on in therapy depends on collaborating with your patient (including perhaps family members and carers) and working out what will be most functionally and socially useful. These goals should be achievable but must aim high enough to motivate the individual.

Unfortunately, goal setting can be particularly complex for people living with a progressively deteriorating disease. Goals are intended to demonstrate some change, yet this is difficult for progressive communication difficulties as no change can be an indicator of success in itself. So considering very carefully what difference intervention will achieve will guide goal setting.

Patients may have very particular ideas about what their current needs are, whilst others may not. Talking to patients about goal setting can be challenging and it is useful to have some ideas of how to support patients in this process. Croot et al. (2009) stresses the importance of preparing patients with progressive conditions for the future in these discussions. This may include setting goals that anticipate future needs, introduce communication aids and working on strategies for the communication partners.

References

Barnes, M.P. (2003) Principles of neurological rehabilitation. *J Neurol. Neurosurg. Psychiatry* **74**, iv3–iv4.

Bier, N., Macoir, J., Gagnon, L., Van der Linden, M., Louveaux, S., & Desrosiers, J. (2009) Known, lost, and recovered: Efficacy of formal-semantic therapy and spaced retrieval method in a case of semantic dementia. *Aphasiology* **23**(2), 210–235.

Cartwright, J. & Elliott, K.A.E. (2009) Promoting strategic television viewing in the context of progressive language impairment. *Aphasiology* **23**(2), 266–285.

Cherney, L.R., Halper, A.S., Holland, A., & Cole, R. (2008) Computerised script training for aphasia: Preliminary results. *American Journal of Speech Language Pathology* **17**, 19–34.

Croot, K., Nickels, L., Laurence, F., & Manning, M. (2009) Impairment- and activity/participation-directed interventions in progressive language impairment: Clinical and theoretical issues. *Aphasiology* **23**(2), 125–160.

Graham, K.S., Pratt, K.H., & Hodges, J.R. (1998) A reverse temporal gradient for public events in a single case of semantic dementia. *Neurocase: The Neural Basis of Cognition* **4**(6), 461–470.

Guthrie, S. & Harvey, A. (1994) Motivation and its influence on outcome in rehabilitation. *Reviews in Clinical Gerontology* **4**(3), 235–243.

Heredia, C.G., Sage, K., Sage, M.A.L., & Berthier, M.L. (2009) Relearning and retention of verbal labels in a case of semantic dementia. *Aphasiology* **23**(2), 192–209.

Jokel, R., Cupit, J., Rochon, E., & Leonard, C. (2009) Relearning lost vocabulary in nonfluent progressive aphasia with MossTalk Words. *Aphasiology* **23**(2), 175–191.

Kindell, J. & Griffiths, H. (2006) Speech and language therapy intervention for people with Alzheimer's disease. In: K. Bryan & J. Maxim (2006) *Communication Disability in the Dementias*. London: Whurr Publishers.

Locke, E.A., Cartledge, N., & Koeppel, J. (1968) Motivational effects of knowledge of results: A goal-setting phenomenon? *Psychological Bulletin* **70**(6), 474–485.

Papp, K.V., Walsh, S.J., & Snyder, P.J. (2009) Immediate and delayed effects of cognitive interventions in healthy elderly: A review of current literature and future directions. *Alzheimer's Dementia* 5(1), 50–60.

Reid, J. (2012) Talking about outcomes and dementia using talking points to promote meaningful engagement demonstrates the impact of Allied Health Professionals' interventions. *Dementia AHP Approaches* 12(1.2). Downloaded from: http://www.knowledge.scot.nhs.uk/media/CLT/ResourceUploads/4018744/DementiaAHPproachesSeptember%202012.pdf

Royal College of Speech and Language Therapists (2005) Clinical Guidelines. Downloaded from: www.rcslt.org/resources/publications

Schut, H.A. & Stam, H.J. (1994) Goals in rehabilitation teamwork. *Disability and Rehabilitation.* 16(4), 223–226.

Snowden, J.S. and Neary, D. (2002) Relearning of verbal labels in semantic dementia. *Neuropsychologia* 40, 1715-1728.

4 Therapy and management: Language impairments

In the management of progressive diseases, language is an area in which we, as a profession, are really expert, particularly in view of all our experience with non-progressive language difficulties. In fact, much of the research has demonstrated that what applies and has been shown to work in treating people with non-progressive aphasia applies to progressive language difficulties.

This chapter discusses a number of areas that frequently arise when working with patients with progressive language difficulties. By no means can this chapter cover all aspects of language, but it does attempt to provide a useful overview of common areas of concern, with case studies to illustrate how therapy can work.

Single words (naming, word finding and comprehension)

Word-finding difficulties are often the first symptoms noticed by people who are developing progressive language difficulties (Mesulam, 2001 cited by Croot, 2009). And these difficulties can have a significant impact on communication. So how can we help? A small number of studies have investigated the effects of different naming therapies in progressive communication difficulties. But there is a much larger number of studies that have been carried out on this topic in the stroke literature. Croot et al. (2009) advocate that, as clinicians, we should readily consider using the same therapies with the progressive client group as we would with our other patients with aphasia.

Therapy tasks

Naming therapies that are undertaken with patients with progressive neurological disorders, particularly the progressive aphasias, will often directly mirror tasks that might be done with stroke patients. So naming therapies could take the form of simple object to picture matching, single word to object matching or object naming. Semantic or phonological cueing, drilling and semantic feature analysis can support these tasks. The choice or task will depend on the level of language impairment. This is where it is vital that your assessment is thorough, just as it would be if you were working with a patient who has had a stroke or brain injury. In order to plan therapy appropriately you need a working hypothesis of the patient's level of language impairment. This hypothesis will likely reflect the diagnosis the individual has been given. Using a framework such as the psycholinguistic model can assist you in this process. If you can hypothesize a semantic breakdown, therapy could target more semantic-based tasks, whilst a phonological assembly impairment may require you to target more phonologically-based activities.

Patients with semantic variant of Primary Progressive Aphasia (svPPA) will present with an evident semantic impairment (including loss of concept knowledge) and therapy will need to address object knowledge as well as naming. If a client can name an object, but is not sure what it is, there appears to be limited future usage, whereas a patient with difficulties accessing word

Table 4.1 Therapy ideas for single word impairments.

Level of hypothesized impairment	Therapy ideas
Semantic impairment (for example, svPPA, some Alzheimer's patients, some HIV dementia patients, perhaps vascular patients who have had stroke events)	Pairing tasks: matching pictures with (spoken and/or written) names Rehearsing names in a category Object naming (with cueing hierarchy from therapist) Reading names aloud Explanation of semantic attributes of target word/object Conversation relating them to everyday place/use/conversation within patient's life Verbal and gestural training of verbs
Word form (or lexical access) impairment (for example, lv PPA)	Naming (with cueing hierarchy of phonological prompts from therapist) Picture matching task, studying of grapheme/written form
Phonological assembly (for example, navPPA, perhaps vascular dementia who have had stroke events, Korsakof/cerebellar dysfunction)	Phoneme discrimination tasks Repetition/drilling target words with model. Reading aloud and self correcting. Scripting of conversation- see sentence level

form in the lexicon will demonstrate knowledge of object function, and may be able to use this as a strategy to support their verbal expression. Follow-up therapy may need to work on matching words to target objects to improve links between these concepts. When working on phonological impairments, however, therapy is likely to target the word form by addressing phonological awareness and self-monitoring as well as articulation, reinforcing phonological representation through drilling. Table 4.1 give more specific therapy ideas for single word impairments. Table 4.2 also summarizes the following discussion with a list of tips and hints for therapy.

Naming task or functional therapy?

When planning intervention you may need to consider where the actual problem in communication lies. Is it the naming difficulty itself or the consequence of the difficulty in conversation; for example, the fact that conversation stops, thoughts are lost and the patient is unable to complete their train of thought. In this case, teaching a patient a repair or circumlocution strategy may be more valid than drilling the naming tasks. Teaching the strategy is the therapy as opposed to teaching the word meaning. Therapy may focus on using spaced retrieval (see later in this chapter) to remember to describe a name or word. This might be particularly useful for patients with naming difficulties in Alzheimer's dementia, who may be more vulnerable to being distracted by their word finding difficulties.

However, if you do choose to focus on a naming task, you might need to consider if the word itself is the most important target for therapy. Is it more important to be able to name something or know what it is used for? Is it more functional for the patient to know that an apple is called 'apple' or that she can eat it and it tastes good? Perhaps working on semantic attributes is more functional for your patient. I would argue that there are many svPPA patients for whom this is true

Learning methods
Cueing techniques

There are different methods of approaching therapy tasks within a therapy session. The clinician must think very carefully about what is most appropriate when planning therapy. The most commonly-used tasks with progressive patients are probably simple repetition and spaced retrieval methods, although the methods most familiar to speech and language therapists are likely to be cueing hierarchies, which are commonly used with patients with non-progressive language impairments. This requires the therapist to provide a graded sequence of cues to access information, for example providing increasing amounts of semantic and/or phonological information such as phonemes, written letters and then written words. Graded cueing techniques are hypothesized to have increased power to support access to word forms.

Simple repetition

Simple repetition requires the patient to repeat each target item a certain number of times within a session, and often therapists and patients will agree on a target. For example, of the ten repetitions they will aim to get nine correct by the end of the 4-week therapy programme. In this case, the therapist should vary presentation order, as list-like repetition will otherwise result in rote learning. So, for example, the therapist might present the same 24 target items ten times in a 45-minute session, but each time they present the target list, the order is varied.

Spaced retrieval

Spaced retrieval is a memory-training procedure and involves systematic recall of information over longer periods of time. In language therapy tasks, the spaced retrieval method might require patients to recollect target words (when presented with a visual stimulus) with increasing time intervals. These are first of all spaced close enough to ensure learning: 15 seconds, 30 seconds, and one minute. After this, spaces are dictated by the patient's performances. So if they make an error, the therapist returns to the last successful gap they achieved. Spaced retrieval is also considered an errorless learning technique, as the patient's errors are monitored; if a hesitation or error is observed the patient is immediately given the target word before continuing. Gaps are filled with general conversation initially but then with alternating presentation of all items as the session progresses. Errorless learning techniques are considered important to accurate learning for people with dementia, as their ability to self-monitor and correct is often impaired. Bourgeois and Hickey (2009) explain that there are two types of memory: declarative and non-declarative. The declarative memory is conscious and involves the retrieval of facts, whilst non-declarative memory recalls procedural, non-conscious information. Patients who have memory difficulties will probably have deficits of declarative memory (Bourgeois & Hickey, 2009) so they will be unable to self-monitor or correct responses. This also means that errors in new learning should be inhibited if possible, as otherwise inaccurate learning will occur. Spaced retrieval has been shown to work with a large variety of progressive dementias. It has been shown to improve face naming, calendar use, mobile phone use, and naming for patients with Alzheimer's disease and progressive diseases (Bier, Macoir, Gagnon, Van der Linden, et al., 2009).

Choosing therapy targets and vocabulary

Some patients arrive at therapy with self-designed therapy programmes, and this might be a useful starting point to engage and support patients with something they are already achieving. Indeed, many authors give examples of self-generated therapy tasks. Jokel, Cupit, Rochon and Leonard (2009) describe a patient who kept notebooks containing lists of written words that he had difficulty retrieving spontaneously. He listed these words into categories and practised them daily. This is perhaps a useful place to start therapy, as this strategy is already a habitual pattern perhaps related to a lifetime of habits. Indeed, it is often the retired university professor, previously a note taker, who arrives with this strategy in place, or the driver who tape-records words and descriptions and listens to them again and again in the car. These examples also demonstrate and provide evidence that regular and ongoing practice allows relearning and maintenance of word lists in some patients (Heredia, Sage, Sage, & Berthier, 2009). Be aware, however, that this list-like approach can also restrict therapy. When Jokel et al. (2009) explored their patient's word learning further, they found he performed rigidly, reflecting the order in which his lists had been written and learned by rote.

A patient may come to therapy with list-learning strategies. This rote learning approach is a concrete method and will possibly prevent generalisation to other words or carryover to real conversations in these patients. This is in part because learning in the normal, intact brain depends on both hippocampal and anterior temporal structures. The hippocampal area allows for rapid learning whilst the anterior temporal lobe gradually forms representations that are flexible, and consequently allows for generalization. This 'longer term memory store' is supported by cortical structures, which may be more vulnerable to disease processes such as dementia (Heredia et al., 2009). Consequently, patients who suffer damage to the anterior temporal lobe area, typical in svPPA, may under- or over-generalize when they relearn words, appearing concrete in their thinking as they are having to depend more on the hippocampus (Mayberry, Sage, Ehsan & Ralph, 2011). Furthermore, the hippocampus learns through discrete separate events, and requires regular exercise to be maintained (Heredia et al., 2009; Mayberry et al., 2011). So if exercise ceases, the effects of the exercise fade. In short, therapy tasks must continue indefinitely to maintain newly-learned words, and therapists must endeavour to support generalization to conversation.

This reinforces the need for careful choice of therapy tasks and target items. It is most useful to choose items on naming tasks that are images or objects from people's real lives. This will promote more meaningful learning methods, as information will be linked to existing knowledge. It will consequently be more likely to generalize to real conversation outside of therapy and will thereby encourage a certain amount of ongoing practice (Mayberry et al., 2011).

How much practice is required?

As with non-progressive aphasia, for people with progressive language impairment intensive practice has been shown to improve outcomes (Bourgeois & Hickey, 2009). But providing such a service is difficult, particularly with the increasing constraints on our healthcare services. Asking patients to continue practising outside of therapy can be a challenge. Many people will verbally commit to a given therapy programme, but actually doing it can be another story. It seems logical that as much practice as possible is best, and that ongoing practice will maintain learned skills. But is this realistic?

Ongoing practice may suit some of our patients, but for others, encouraging them to take this task on board may simply require some imagination. Sitting down at the table to do 'homework' can be terribly dull for some, whilst for others, who have always had to do some kind of paperwork, it may be perfectly natural. Perhaps asking our patients what they deem is appropriate and acceptable could be more helpful – some may be able to use computer-based therapy tasks that they can continue at home independently. This may also save on time and resources for the initial therapy phase itself. Some might benefit from telephone therapy sessions, or just a verbal prompt on the telephone to remind them. Others might choose to record their therapy tasks in videotaped sessions and use these at home. Some people might wish to involve family members in supporting them with their practice, but be careful in suggesting this as other patients may not wish to involve anybody else.

Most important of all, perhaps, is that the more that therapy can target vocabulary which is real and meaningful for a patient (that they link to their own environment), the more likely these concepts will be maintained. This may be achieved during therapy by using objects and talking about them in the patient's own home. Other strategies might include encouraging patients and their carers to store things in the same place, follow the same routine, go to the same place for shopping and other daily activities and being loyal to brands. These strategies in turn can promote carryover to real conversations. Heredia et al. (2009) suggest that carryover to conversation creates an informal maintenance practice plan, negating the need for more formal ongoing therapy practice.

Table 4.2 Quick and simple tips for therapies when planning single-word therapies.

Let your hypothesis guide your therapy task.
Work out what will be most useful for patients – the words themselves or strategies?
Consider learning strategies – are you going to used cued learning, drilling or spaced retrieval methods?
Support patients to select their own target words or vocabulary.
Use the patient's own objects (or photographs of these).
Do therapy in a patient's own home where possible, or in a relevant meaningful location.
Can you justify ongoing rehearsal?
If you are encouraging some kind of maintenance programme, be innovative.

What does the evidence show us?

There is indeed evidence that shows the therapy approaches described in this chapter can improve and maintain naming and word finding for patients with various dementias. Unfortunately, there are some barriers to finding and examining the literature in this area. Primarily, it is the diagnostic terminology used by researchers that can make this tricky. Often authors will use different diagnostic criteria (such as the features of the different primary progressive aphasias) and terminology (such as using semantic dementia) or use more generic inclusion criteria (for example, they may not differentiate between types of dementia at all, and simply include anyone with a 'dementia' diagnosis). There has recently been more agreement on the use of this terminology, as discussed in Chapter 2, which should make it easier to search for evidence that applies to specific patient groups such as svPPA versus navPPA. Having said that, the literature here will be slanted to the Primary Progressive Aphasias, particularly the semantic variant, as this has been the focus of most research studies focusing on language therapies.

There are, however, a number of therapy programmes that have demonstrated improvements in naming for patients with Alzheimer's disease. Clare et al. (1999, cited by Graham, Pratt, & Hodges, 1999) demonstrated that errorless learning in face-naming tasks with ongoing practice allowed a patient to relearn the names of the members of his bowls club. This is a similar approach used in much of the research for therapy with patients with svPPA.

Some of the earliest examples of investigations into therapy options for patients with progressive language impairments have come from and still do come from retrospective case studies. Some of these studies highlight and explore programmes that patients had developed for themselves and that seemed to successfully improve and maintain their naming skills. One such example is described by Graham et al. (1999). They describe how a patient with semantic dementia (DM), previously a surgical consultant, had developed written lists, accompanied by written definitions, pictures from a picture dictionary and photos for face naming, which he practised daily. He used these lists by covering the target words and attempting to name the descriptions or image. They tested his list learning and found that he was able to improve his ability in new categories of word generation by practising new lists (particularly if they were practised in category order). They also found that when he stopped practising his scores deteriorated. They hypothesized that his practice method of linking semantic and word form information, his seemingly errorless learning style and his perhaps milder degree of anomia contributed to his performance.

Since then, a number of therapy programmes such as the one described by Jokel, Rochon and Leonard (2006) have shown that patients with svPPA can benefit from structured naming therapy tasks. Jokel et al. (2006) used patient-selected words and set up a daily home practice regime where pictures were paired with written, phonological and semantic information (the patient was required to name the target, read the name aloud and read personally-relevant information). The programme was completed six days per week, for 30 minutes each day, over a course of two weeks. The effects of this programme did not generalize to other items, but were maintained one month later. Some of these benefits were still evident six months later.

Many authors discuss the impact of dosage of therapy in their investigations.

Bier et al. (2009) describe a therapy programme for a patient with semantic dementia. They delivered a series of six sessions where they compared using simple repetition (three sessions) to spaced retrieval (three sessions) for naming and object descriptions. Both methods resulted in improvements, with no specific differences between the two. The authors hypothesized that perhaps the most important thing is the number of attempts made at the target within one session. Whilst both approaches resulted in improvements, these were not maintained at five weeks post treatment.

Other authors attempt to highlight the value of aspects of therapy that successfully promote maintenance of therapy effects. Heredia et al. (2009) described a therapy programme for a patient with semantic dementia. They demonstrated a therapy task targeting 28 words, where each item was first presented as a picture followed by the picture paired with the written label. Therapy required the patient to name the picture, and if unable to name it, to turn to the labelled picture and read the name aloud. The patient practised this every day for one month in the same order. Results showed that the gains made immediately after therapy were maintained up to six months later. The researchers highlighted that this patient was required to practise for one month, whilst many other studies examined results after only two weeks. This highlights the importance of the dose effect in this study. Heredia et al. (2009) also emphasized that improvements on word use were also generalized to spontaneous speech. They felt it was this that contributed to maintenance, by creating an informal practice regime. And by talking about the items outside of therapy the patient was possibly more able to link words to the real home environment and actual functional use of the target object words in daily activities. Heredia et al. (2009) hypothesize that this carryover to conversation made the therapy material more 'meaningful'.

The use of more cost-effective therapies that minimize expensive face-to-face clinician time has also been explored with this client group in the literature. Jokel et al. (2009) describe a computer-based system with three modules called Mosstalk word (www.mosstalk.com), which uses either preprogrammed exercises or custom-made tasks tailored to the needs of individual participants. Jokel et al. (2009) investigated the use of this system with 'nonfluent progressive aphasic' patients. However, in their description of the individuals' impairments, the participants demonstrated intact articulation and grammar but poor repetition and sentence comprehension as well as anomia. These patients likely presented with an lvPPA. This difference in the use of diagnostic terminology reflects the difference across institutions and makes it much more difficult to analyze the literature for what might work with our own clients. The researchers used a cued naming module with written initial letter and written whole word cues (the hypothesis being that these individuals had difficulties accessing phonological word forms). Pictures were randomly presented on a screen (from the target 20 items developed in conjunction with the patient), and no feedback was given. When the patient was unable to name the item, the first letter cue was provided. If this did not cue a response then the whole word was presented; if the patient was unable to say it, then the clinician produced a model for the patient to repeat. The patient was always given all cues and asked to repeat the word, even if they were successful. Jokel et al. (2009) suggested that key to this therapy approach for naming is the requirement that the patient state the name out loud, as it is this that facilitates better maintenance of treatment effects. They also emphasized that involving the patient actively in therapy stimulates a deeper processing and results in longer-lasting effects. The results showed patients made gains on all treated items for up to four weeks post treatment. This was not maintained six months later. And there was no impact at all on untreated words. However, patients did demonstrate improved syntactic production immediately post treatment, although this also declined at six months post treatment. Interestingly, those participants who were able to commit to more intense therapy (e.g. more frequently per week and at least three times per week) were able to make bigger, quicker gains compared to those who could only commit to one or two sessions per week. Jokel et al. (2009) highlighted that there are limitations to using computer-based programs and explained that patients are often reluctant to practise independently, thereby defeating the purpose of the task design. They also reported that home practice using this system does require occasional clinician guidance.

More recently, there has been some focus on other variants of progressive aphasia, including navPPA, in the research literature (Henry, Meese, Truong, et al., 2012). These researchers examined the effect of oral reading practice on the production of multisyllabic words when read aloud. They also examined how this generalized to untrained speech behaviours. Text was chosen jointly by the patient and clinician, and was read aloud by the patient until a word was incorrectly produced. If this was a multisyllabic word it was then underlined and divided into syllables so it could be produced syllable by syllable, and then as an entire word until it was stated correctly. Reading would then recommence from the start of the sentence in which the error had occurred. Treatment sessions were held once a week for 12 weeks and supplemented by home practice five times per week. The researchers found that the patient was able to read untrained text aloud with fewer errors and improved success in self-corrections after therapy. They also found improved speech production in repetition of long sentences and trisyllabic words. They found that the patient's speech sound errors in connected speech probes had not deteriorated any further a year after treatment, although they did observe a worsening in phonetic distortions, speech rate and number of pauses. Henry et al. (2012) emphasize that the success of this treatment approach was partly attributable to the participant's ability to accurately self-detect errors. This could limit the application of this technique with other patients who do not have such accurate self-monitoring skills.

Finally Farrajota, Maruta, Maroco et al. (2012) have attempted to branch out from case studies to a controlled intervention trial. They examined the effectiveness of speech and language therapy for a group of patients with PPA and compared them to a control group not receiving therapy. The authors do not specify what therapy the participants received other than that they attended weekly sessions of up to 60 minutes focusing on a multimodal stimulation approach targeting different exercises such as picture naming, picture description, comprehension tasks and reading and writing as well as conversational strategies. All patients in the study had been diagnosed with PPA, but no specific information was provided on whether different variants were treated differently. There are evident limitations to this study and its application to clinical practice, yet this research did demonstrate that patients receiving therapy intervention tended to decline less than those not receiving therapy intervention.

There is much more research to be done in this area, both academically and clinically, but already we can apply what the research tells us to our daily practice.

Case study 1: Mr B

Mr B is a 59-year-old gentleman who came to the outpatient service with a diagnosis of primary progressive aphasia of the semantic variant. He reported that his mother also had dementia, having been diagnosed with Alzheimer's disease. She now lived in a nursing home local to his home. Mr B attended the appointment with his wife. Both Mr and Mrs B still worked, and lived at home with one of their two young adult children. Mr B owned his own building business, and still regularly attended social events with friends. However, the couple reported that Mr B was experiencing increasing difficulties thinking of words and understanding some words. This was causing a particular problem for him at work, where he would find it difficult to order materials or hand people tools they asked for. On assessment, using the comprehensive aphasia test and parts of the PALPA, Mr B presented with both single word comprehension and naming difficulties, although naming was more impaired than comprehension.

Mr B reported he had already started putting together a tape recording using a dictaphone he had at home. On this tape he recorded words he felt he was 'forgetting' and the dictionary definition of this word. He would then listen to these words whilst driving in his car. In agreement with his therapist, Mr B first of all went home and took photos of all his tools, and then visited his local warehouse where he photographed all the materials he routinely purchased. He then brought these photos to therapy where he explained the function of all the tools and identified the names (with assistance) of all the photos. The therapist then produced a book of cards using these photos, with the object names printed on the reverse. The patient and the therapist planned a set of six sessions where they completed two tasks. The first task required Mr B to name each picture (at random), read the name written on the reverse and describe its function and relevance to work. If he hesitated or was unable to name the item he was encouraged to turn the picture over immediately and read the word aloud. The second task required Mr B to listen to a target word given by the therapist, and find it from the set of photos (this task was divided into two categories: materials/tools). Mr B was asked to practise the first task at home each evening. After about half the sessions had been completed Mr B stated he felt confident about continuing this task independently at home but that therapy was difficult to attend due to work commitments. Mr B reported he felt therapy had helped and he planned to continue at home independently. He also reported he had labelled all his tools, and had spoken to his colleagues about his difficulties. He requested one further session to complete a tape recording of the target vocabulary, with a recorded definition. Mr B and the therapist worked together to develop a tape recording; modifying his method somewhat by leaving an extended pause between the word and the definition allowing him the opportunity to provide an online answer (when listening to the tape) before the answer was given.

Mr B revisited the clinic approximately four months later, stating that he had continued the therapy programme irregularly (due to work commitments) but that he didn't feel his 'tools' or 'materials' vocabulary had deteriorated. However, he did report deterioration in other areas of language, and periods of low mood. Consequently, he was referred to the psychologist for a period of intervention. He continued to attend speech and language therapy sessions at regular intervals for approximately two and half years.

Examples of target vocabulary for Mr B

Hammer	It's a tool to bang in nails
Spirit level	You use it to check how straight your work is, like a shelf
Wood saw	You use it to saw through wood
Hack saw	You use it to saw through metal
Jab saw	You use it for precise sawing
Orbital sander	An electric powered tool, you use it to sand wood
Sheet sander	An electric powered tool, you use it for sanding larger flat surfaces like walls and doors
Planer	An electric powered tool, you use it for planing wood to size
Angle grinder	An electric powered tool, you use it for cutting tiles or stone, and sometimes steel
Cold chisel	You use it for cutting steel, brick and concrete by hand
Wood chisel	You use it for cutting, carving and shaving wood by hand

Using words and sentences

Working on single words is one way of structuring therapy but, as we all well know, conversation is not made up of a series of single words – it is made up of sentences. And sentences can be particularly difficult for people living with some variants of progressive language impairment. As its name suggests, the nonfluent agrammatic variant of primary progressive aphasia is particularly characterized by agrammatic speech. However, sentences can easily be interrupted by word-finding difficulties that distract individuals such that they are unable to continue the sentence or the topic at hand. This is common to many variants of dementia, including patients with Alzheimer's dementia and those with the logopenic variant of primary progressive aphasia. As with single word-based therapies there is much we can share and learn from the non-progressive language impairments here. Unfortunately, however, the evidence for these therapies in the progressive language disorders literature is scarce.

Therapy tasks

As with single word-based therapies you must understand the nature of the sentence breakdown in order to judge which would be the most appropriate therapy task. If a patient produces sentences that are grammatically sound but nonfluent and empty of content, they may be struggling with word generation. This may mean patients could benefit from single word-based therapies to support their sentence level skills. Working on nouns and verb meanings could support patients in maintaining their repertoire of words and thus the content of the sentences they produce. Sentence scripting and drilling may also improve fluency for specific sentences and phrases.

A patient who produces sentences which are agrammatic or limited to very simply structured sentences may also benefit from scripting and drilling therapies. Relearning sentence rules through teaching sentence structures could also help. However, when we look to the evidence for single word therapies it seems that patients with progressive language impairment lack many of the skills necessary to learn a rule and generalize it to unlearned words. Yet these patients can learn and maintain specific context-relevant language. So learning a sentence 'rule' and applying it to as yet unplanned sentences may be unrealistic. In comparison, using principles of scripting (choosing specific sentences relevant to the patient's real life, that can be practised daily to ensure maintenance) is perhaps the more realistic approach.

As we discussed in Chapter 3, patients will often direct the clinician to what they would prefer to work on when planning therapy. Patients may tell their clinicians that they just want to be able to converse with a certain group of friends, or talk at length on a certain topic. This is where sentence-based drilling might work best. However, it is difficult to discuss conversation here without thinking of the conversation partners themselves. Conversation partners are considered in more detail in Chapter 6. In this section, we will continue to discuss therapy approaches that can improve sentence production. Table 4.3 summarises these therapy ideas.

Table 4.3 Therapy ideas for sentence and word impairments.

Level of impairment:	Suggested therapy tasks
Word-finding difficulties (svPPA, lvPPA, Alzheimer's disease and perhaps vascular dementia)	Single word therapies, particularly gesture-based therapy targeting verb generation/tense markers (past and future) Scripting and drilling of target phrases, sentences and topics
Agrammatic speech (navPPA)	Stimulation through reading and auditory comprehension tasks (where patient listens to or reads sentences or paragraphs and answers questions related to content) Re-teaching sentence structures in formal therapy where the patient has to generate written or spoken sentences to picture stimuli Scripting and drilling of target phrases, sentences and topics Reading aloud and self-monitoring (see Chapter 3)

Gestures

This type of therapy may be seen as promoting more compensatory strategies to support communication rather than improve verbal language skills. However, there is much discussion in the research that suggests gestures can improve access to word forms by increasing stimulation to the pre-frontal cortex, so priming access to word forms and assisting in word form retrieval. It may be considered intuitive as we find ourselves waving our hands around to try to show what we mean if we are unable to recall the words, so why shouldn't it work for people with communication difficulties. Scheider et al. (1996) describe a detailed therapy approach that taught the use of pantomime-type gesture for nouns, verbs and tense markers in target structures in sentences. These skills were developed in the clinic alongside independent home-based practice using pictures of the targeted gestures.

Scripting

Script knowledge includes understanding, remembering and recalling the temporal organization of events in routine activity (Cherney, Halper, Holland & Cole, 2008). The principles of scripting are based in the instance theory of automatization (Logan, 1988, cited by Cherney et al., 2008). This theory indicates that some highly routinised tasks or skills are specific context-bound driven memories. By this rationale, some things are better not broken down but practised as a whole. This therapy approach reflects the theory described previously in single word therapies by Bourgeois and Hickey (2009). They hypothesize that people with dementia, particularly progressive language difficulties, have difficulties with declarative memories, affecting skills such as self-monitoring, whilst non-declarative memories are generally considered more automatic and very situation specific and are consequently less impaired. In theory, an approach such as scripting harnesses a patient's strengths by employing their generally more preserved comprehension, recall of events and ability to function otherwise well in a real everyday activity.

Scripts are designed to enable a patient to learn specific phrases related to a specific situation. They involve intensive drilling practice using a cueing hierarchy over a number of sessions. Drilling is often achieved through repeated oral reading or computer-based systems. Audrey Holland has written much on this topic in the non-progressive literature. In fact, the process for script writing has been standardized by the Center for Aphasia Research at the Rehabilitation Institute of Chicago and, more recently, has been developed into a software tool (Cherney et al., 2008).

Holland advocates for patients' rights to be able to 'tell a story' and participate in personally relevant conversational activities. And this is just what scripting can do. To develop an appropriate script the speech and language therapist and the patient need to create an individualized script together. By considering the person's communication needs in a detailed conversational interview (similar to the goal-focused needs discussion described in Chapter 3), the clinician and the patient can identify useful situations for which to draft scripts. Holland (2008) highlights that people often like to speak about topics to do with their illness story and their family, and want common social phrases associated with everyday situations such as using the telephone, ordering in a coffee shop, and so on. Case Study 2 includes a good example of the type of scripted conversation that could be worked on.

There are however, some limitations to this drilling technique – particularly that generalization to other sentences or across situations is unlikely. This therapy approach may not always seem that useful to us as clinicians as these are scripts that can only be used in a finite number of situations, but it can provide the opportunity for people to maintain part of their identity through sharing anecdotes and stories.

Other clinicians have interpreted this principle in other ways and, rather than relearning entire stories, they promote the learning of a predictable conversation, using a predictable set of questions which can be flexed to different themes. Such approaches do require support from the conversation partner, and has been described as scaffolding by some. Cartwright and Elliott (2009) developed a conversational support targeting television viewing (described in more detail below). The form followed a structure with predictable questions and topics. In some ways, this model of therapy incorporates principles from both more formal therapeutic principles of sentence comprehension tasks and relearning of sentence rules, where patients are asked to listen and summarize an episode and then discuss the episode using a pre-learned structure. This approach also allows for carryover by attaching this conversation to a specific activity, which happens on a regular, if not daily, basis.

What does the evidence show us?

The evidence in the area of sentence level therapies for progressive language disorders is scant at best. Authors have described some exploratory case studies, retrospectively. This type of study can also inform our practice. But again, we can look to the non-progressive literature for support. It isn't within the realm of this chapter to comment on the literature available for non-progressive sentence level therapies. And, indeed, there are many excellent and easily accessible texts available on this topic. The following describes just a handful of studies that have been done with progressive language impairments, mostly with people with PPA.

Murray (1998) published a case study describing a client with non-fluent primary progressive aphasia and the various treatment approaches used over a number of years. The first phase of treatment included two sentence level tasks. The first involved listening to and reading sentences or paragraphs and answering questions about them. The second required the patient to generate spoken and written sentences using specified sentence structures (subject is/are verb) to describe action pictures. Therapy resulted in significant improvements in accuracy on all the tasks, but no carryover to everyday conversation. Murray then goes on to describe further therapy strategies as the patient's condition worsened. This is quite different to treatment designed by Henry et al. (2012), which focused on self-monitoring phonological errors when reading aloud for a patient with navPPA, described in detail under the single word therapies. Henry et al. did find improvements in fluency in sentence production but did not focus on the agrammatic impairment itself. This illustrates how different therapy approaches can impact on sentence production in different ways in the same person. Considering which area is causing the biggest problem can guide you in this choice.

Other, quite different, approaches to sentence therapies have also been anecdotally described in the literature; such as that reported by Scheider et al. (1996). They describe a therapy approach that taught the use of pantomimed-type gesture for nouns, verbs and tense markers in target structures in sentences. These skills were developed over 18 sessions, alongside home-based practice using pictures of the target gestures. They found improvements in target words and gestures carried over to conversation and story recall and patients were able to use trained sentences in story recall. Unfortunately, this wasn't maintained three months later, and only the gestures continued to be used, not the verbal targets.

Scripting as described by Audrey Holland has received no attention in the progressive aphasia literature to date, as far as I am aware. In general, the focus of this therapy approach has been with non-fluent, non-progressive aphasias. Scripting therapy with these patients generally focuses on developing and then training specific sentences in a cued massed practice system. Cued mass practice requires continued drilling until patients achieve over 90% accuracy. The results of this research demonstrate that patients can achieve improved fluency in sentence production for specific phrases, but there is no carryover to other items (Youmans, Holland, Munoz & Bourgeois, 2005). Holland has also recently started focusing on the use of a computer-based virtual therapist to support this intensive training system which may also be useful for patients with progressive aphasias (Cherney et al., 2008).

However, some researchers have described similar principles to scripting with progressive language impairments. The idea of 'telling a story' that is central to Audrey Holland's approach to scripting has been explored in other ways by other researchers. One example of this might be described as using storytelling techniques and conversational guides for functional situations. Cartwright and Elliott (2009) developed a therapy programme targeting television viewing. As dementia advances, our patients could become frailer and therefore more housebound, perhaps meaning that they spend more time watching television than previously. Cartwright and Elliott (2009) highlighted that patients with language impairment will inevitably find that the listening and comprehension involved in television viewing becomes more problematic as their difficulties progress. The researchers urge that, as clinicians, we might not be maximizing the potential neuroprotective abilities of this tool. They suggest that by increasing the social and cognitive demands surrounding TV viewing the neuroprotective qualities of this leisure pursuit can be enhanced, thereby perhaps slowing the rate of neurodegenerative decline. Although this does not immediately appear to be a therapy targeting sentences, the therapy programme used in the study itself does. Cartwright and Elliott (2009) describe a 10-week group format, where clients with progressive language difficulties associated with various dementias attend with their partners. At each session patients are taught a glossary of TV-related vocabulary such as 'episode=session', as well as viewing an episode of a popular TV programme. They pause the programme regularly and discuss and summarize the episode allowing opportunities for questions. They then discuss and debate the episode, using and completing a form to summarize the entire show and guide conversation. The form follows a structure that guides conversation with predictable questions and topics. The participants are then asked to do the same task at least twice with their partners at home each week. Cartwright and Elliott (2009) describe an improvement in the abilities of all the patients to recall information about the 'television story' in conversation. They also report improvements in the ability of patients to understand and answer questions on the target topic in conversation. Although this is not strictly an impairment-based therapy, this approach to therapy demonstrates how to develop conversational frameworks that are repeatedly used in therapy situations until they become predictable and scripted. It also highlights how impairment-based therapy can be built around functional, regularly encountered situations in order to maximize usefulness and carryover.

> **Case Study 2: Mr C**
>
> Mr C was a 64-year-old gentleman who lived at home, on his own. Mr C was diagnosed with non-fluent progressive aphasia by his local memory service. They referred him to community services regarding concerns about how he was managing at home. His mother lived in a local nursing home and had been diagnosed with dementia some time before. Mr C's description of his mother's difficulties suggested she might have experienced a similar decline in communication to his before she developed more significant mobility difficulties. Mr C had a previous history of anxiety and depression, and had been his mother's carer until she moved into residential care some five years previously. He reported that it was around three years later that he noticed his own communication difficulties developing, and consequently his uncle suggested that he have them investigated.
>
> Mr C was quite socially isolated, with no family or friends close by. He enjoyed photography, and was keen to socialize but wasn't sure how to re-engage socially now that he no longer had to care for his mother at home. On assessment, he presented with non-fluent speech, with lots of phonological errors and significant effort and groping at times when speaking. He also demonstrated agrammatic sentence structure in expression. However, he described himself as a chatterbox and a joker who enjoyed conversation and company. The multidisciplinary team working with Mr C supported him to access local social groups, particularly a photography group. Mr C requested a 'story' to explain his difficulties with communication. As a result, Mr C and his speech and language therapist decided to script a monologue and a series of social conversational phrases in preparation for attending his local men's group. Mr C required a lot of support to practise these phrases and had additional sessions with the rehabilitation assistant as well as the speech and language therapist. Mr C and the therapist also discussed the idea of creating a video of the therapist doing the exercises to support him at home, although Mr C eventually decided against this as he did not own a working video player or equivalent. Mr C went on to attend the photography group and used his 'story' at the first session he

attended. Although we had scripted the monologue Mr C decided to read the script aloud on the day. He consequently reported significantly more confidence in attempting any kind of conversation (Mr C preferred a total communication approach) including the use of a couple of communication aid cards he had developed with the therapist.

Example of Mr C's scripts

My 'story'

My name is Mr C. I have a type of disease called progressive aphasia. It makes talking difficult. I am here today with my photos. I have always loved taking photos. I wanted to share them with you all. The photos are from all over the local area. They are things I have seen. And they are things I liked.

Conversational phrases

> Patient's script: *How are you?*
>
> Example of other's likely response: Good, how are you?
>
> Patient's script: *Well, thank you. What have you been up to this week?*
>
> Example of other's likely response: I saw my family and went bowling.
>
> Patient's script: *How is your family?*
>
> Example of other's likely response: Good – the usual. What have you been up to?
>
> Patient's script: *Not much. I did some photography.*
>
> Example of other's likely response: Sounds good, what did you photograph?
>
> Patient's script: *The fields at the bottom of my road. They are beautiful.*
>
> Example of other's likely response: I bet.

Reading, writing and communication aids

Some research suggests that reading skills can be more preserved than spoken language in patients with progressive language impairments, particularly progressive aphasia (Papp, Walsh & Snyder, 2009). There is also some suggestion that reading and writing skills are consequently more amenable to improvements with therapy exercise. Importantly, reading and writing can serve a greater overall purpose for this client group, by facilitating access to conversation when verbal skills are not effective. This is perhaps what makes them so precious in the long term and, consequently, worth investing time and therapy in. Indeed, many patients with progressive diseases, particularly those with memory difficulties, may be able to use communication aids or total communication strategies well into the moderate or advanced stages of their condition. This may include writing single words or phrases alongside gesture and spoken words in a conversation, or writing notes to aid memory or reading information from a memory book or talking mats system to support conversation.

Table 4.4 Therapy ideas for reading, writing and communication aids.

Level of impairment	Suggested therapy task
Surface dyslexic errors: difficulties with reading and spelling of familiar words with phonological plausible errors due to deficits in the orthographic lexicon – svPPA	Spell-study-spell programmes Functional approaches to writing tasks such as using spell check or letter frameworks
Phonological dyslexic errors: difficulties reading and spelling unfamiliar words using sounding-out methods due to deficits in the phonology-orthography conversion system –Alzheimer's disease, lvPPA and navPPA	Reading aloud and self correcting (see evidence in 'Single words' section of this chapter)
Either of the above + / conversation breakdown due to language or cognitive impairment	Communication aids Training in the use of total communication Lo-tech aids such as communication books and Talking Mats Hi-tech aids such as computer tablets (i-pads).

This section discusses therapy approaches that target improvements in both spelling and writing. The use of communication aids is well described and constantly being updated for people with progressive diseases. Consequently, this text will not explore a vast number of these options. However, we do describe a couple of examples that are perhaps particularly relevant for the dementia population. See Table 4.4 for further therapy ideas.

It is also relevant to re-emphasize the importance of assessing and understanding an individual's reading and writing skills for communication aid selection. Being able to judge if a patient can read large or small type, single words or sentences, as well as knowing the level of dyslexic impairment, will guide symbol choice and consequently choice of communication aid. It is also valuable when developing this plan to consider who the person will be communicating with. There are some guides to assessing and developing appropriate communication aid devices on the market such as the Social Networks package developed by Blackstone and Hunt-Berg (2012).

Reading and writing

If you are considering working on improving or maintaining reading and writing skills, you must seriously consider why you are doing this. Is this person still working and/or using writing as part of their daily activities, for example, writing letters, reports, emails or invoices? And, if so, what kind of errors are they making; are the errors word errors related to their semantic knowledge or spelling errors related to true progressive dyslexia? Will a spell check do? Or is therapy actually going to be useful?

There are very few suggestions or therapy approaches that have been described to support reading and writing for people with progressive language difficulties or dementia. So, much of what we have already described in this chapter will apply to reading and writing, namely that therapy approaches for non-progressive aphasias will often be applicable to people with progressive conditions. However, it is unusual to find many patients with dementia who have a burning concern to work on their reading and writing skills. The only instance that I can truly think of is where an older lady with Alzheimer's disease and phonological dyslexia wanted to work on her ability to write letters to old friends in another country with whom she still kept in contact. In this example, we developed a letter-writing framework. We wrote out an agreed basic skeleton of what she would typically include in a letter, with spaces where she could insert appropriate words. For these spaces we created word lists so she was able to choose which words she would prefer to include from the list and copy them in. She often needed help from her husband to identify which words to insert, but she enjoyed being able to complete the majority of the task independently. This is a very functional solution to a writing difficulty and mirrors many of the principles we have mentioned in previous parts of this chapter as it was a highly specific contextualized task with a narrow range of words chosen by the patient herself, and consequently more salient.

Papp et al. (2009) do provide an example of therapy for writing difficulties for people with progressive aphasia in a case study. They report on a written therapy programme that focused on a spell-study-spell system. They describe a patient who presented with a progressive dyslexia characterized by phonologically plausible errors, such as reading /sew/ as /sue/. This patient also presented with difficulties in longer words and no significant differences between oral and written spelling. This suggests intact phonological skills, but difficulties in graphemic buffering and in the orthographic lexicon typical of surface dyslexia in svPPA. They describe using a procedure where the patient was required to spell each word and then study the correct form, whilst the presenter repeated the word and named each letter. Finally, the patient then attempted to spell each word again, until it was spelled correctly (or three times). They also described using a homework task where the patient was asked to copy a word 10 times, then turn the page and write it from memory before checking it and studying it carefully.

Henry et al. (2012) have recently described a novel therapy approach in a case study of an individual who was making speech errors and who had been diagnosed with navPPA. These researchers examined the effect of oral reading practice on production of multisyllabic words read aloud. Text was chosen jointly by the patient and clinician and then read aloud by the patient until a word was incorrectly produced. If this was a multisyllabic word it was then underlined and divided into syllables so it could be produced syllable by syllable, and then as an entire word until it was stated correctly. Reading would then recommence from the start of the sentence in which the error had occurred. This therapy practice was continued by the patient outside of therapy sessions once it had been established that the person could reliably self-monitor and recognize errors. Although this therapy approach was specifically designed to treat spoken errors it could also be argued that it targeted reading skills too. However, further research would be required to evidence this as an outcome.

Communication aids

Both expert clinicians and the literature support the use of alternative communication for people with progressive language impairments. Clinicians have described using many innovative methods including written or pictorial aids, gestures, sign or technology-based solutions. This may include communication books, boards and communication cards. Teaching total communication including drawing, writing, gesture and intonation can also be valuable. In addition, adaptive equipment such as a personal alarm or a computer-based aid have been found to be useful. Most of these approaches will incorporate a degree of writing or reading and some clinicians may advocate that working on reading or writing to support access to specific aids will be most useful. This might include working on symbol recognition to access hi-tech aids, or single word recognition for lo-tech aids.

Most recently, there has been an increased discussion about the positive impact a tablet computer or phone can have for people with various types of dementia (SIG Psycho-geriatric, 2012). In fact, I have found that many clients, even those who have never before used a computer, work well with many of the tablet computers available on the market, particularly the widely available Apple products (such as an i-pad, i-touch or i-phone). This tool is extremely flexible and many of its features, such as the camera, lend themselves well to supporting communication. For example, they enable people with svPPA to take photos of family members and events they attended to support conversation, to photograph the food items they might need before going to find these in the supermarket, or using many of the available apps (both free or not). The apps available are constantly being updated and the best advice I can give is to search the app-stores to see what is available.

There are also a number of lo-tech tools that have been developed and modified for use with people with dementia. Talking Mats is a low technology communication framework developed at the University of Stirling, in Scotland. It is a simple system of picture symbols that are placed on a textured mat in a particular order to allow people to discuss and indicate their views. Murphy, Oliver and Cox (2010) describe this system in significant detail. They describe sitting down with individuals with dementia in front of a Talking Mat and asking them to place images related to a particular topic onto the mat using a visual scale. For example, if the discussion is around support for daily living the person can place pictorial images or words related to different activities on a scale, rating them as "Things I can do on my own, things I am unsure about, and things I need support with" (see Figure 4.1). The recommendation is that the conversation should then be recorded by taking a photo of the completed mat, ultimately acting as a permanent record and a memory aid for future conversations. There is some research examining the use of Talking Mats with people with dementia, which will be described later in this chapter. However, there has been a significant emphasis on using the Talking Mats tool as a support in decision-making, and this will be discussed in more detail in Chapter 7.

What does the evidence say?

The literature on reading and writing therapies is not only extremely limited for adults with dementia but often is more opinion based than research based. There is some evidence from case studies that suggests more formal writing therapies can have a positive effect. There is also some more robust evidence examining the use of some specific communication aids, particularly Talking Mats, for people with dementia. However, I wonder if this is an area where

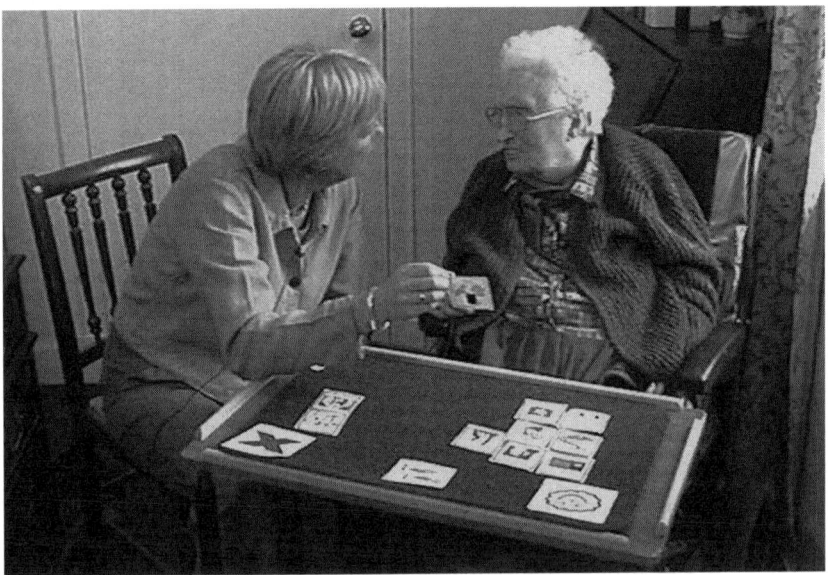

Figure 4.1 Using Talking Mats to support conversation with people with dementia. (Reproduced by permission of J. Murphy, www.talkingmats.com.)

there will be a significant increase in research literature in the near future, especially as technological advances mean that computer tablets and apps are becoming more affordable and accessible. But do not let this put you off: just because there is no research evidence doesn't mean it won't work for your patient. Being innovative and reactive to patient needs is part of being evidence based. The following briefly summarizes what little evidence there is in the research literature.

In the above section on written therapies, Papp et al.'s spell-study-spell programme for surface dyslexia was described in some detail. Papp et al. (2009) describe using a programme where the patient is required to spell each word, study the correct form, whilst the presenter repeats the word and names each letter. Finally the patient then attempts to spell it again, until it is spelled correctly. Part of this programme also involves a homework task where the patient is asked to copy a word 10 times, and then write it from memory before checking it. They report that the first system demonstrated an improvement in performance on individual items. In comparison, the second approach demonstrated no improvements in performance on spelling words. However, the second task did support maintenance of learned spellings, where other unpractised words continued to deteriorate.

In terms of communication aids, there is a strongly-held opinion in the speech and language therapy community that communication aids can be useful for most patients with progressive conditions. Much of the literature relevant to people with dementia and primary progressive aphasia is anecdotal at this stage. Cress and King, for example (1999, cited by Papp et al.), describe teaching a patient with dementia to use symbols on a communication board, whilst Pattee et al. (2006), cited by Papp et al., 2009) report how one of their patients with PPA demonstrated improvements in using a spelling-led communication aid. They also highlight this patient's preference in using a spelling-led aid versus a speech-based device. These examples stress the variety of communication aid options available and the importance of considering patient preferences in choosing such aids. Not everyone likes to communicate in the same style in verbal conversation; similarly, they may have different likes and dislikes about communication aids.

Murphy and her colleagues have conducted a number of studies into the use of Talking Mats with people with dementia. Murphy, Gray and Cox (2007) conducted a larger-scale research study into the use of Talking Mats to support communication between unfamiliar listeners and patients with dementia. They used Talking Mats in conversations to examine how 31 people at different stages of dementia felt about their lives. The researchers determined effectiveness by examining video clips of conversations and rating how much the person with dementia understood, the degree of engagement, ability to stay on topic and degree to which the listener could understand the person with dementia. They found that people could communicate more effectively using Talking Mats compared to unstructured or semi-structured conversations. They also found that patients produced more reliable information when using Talking Mats than structured conversation, when information was compared to real life events. Murphy et al. (2007) did make some practical recommendations about using Talking Mats that included the need for personalized images if necessary, and that symbols need to be simple with large text. Finally, they highlighted that some participants may need support in placing pictures.

More recently, Murphy et al. (2010) conducted a similar research study but with 18 couples, again comparing the use of Talking Mats to 'normal' verbal conversations. People with dementia and their carers were asked to discuss if they were managing or needing support in four aspects of daily living: personal care, getting around, housework and activities. The researchers examined the effectiveness of these conversations using a similar method as previously and found that patients were more engaged in conversations using Talking Mats than in normal conversations. People with dementia were able to keep on track and perseverate less. They demonstrated more confidence and were often able to take control of the mat. The researcher examining the video was better able to understand the person with dementia when using a Talking Mat. The researchers also observed an improved conversational balance between couples using Talking Mats when compared to 'normal conversations'. Murphy et al. (2010) found that carers also felt more listened to in Talking Mats discussions, and attributed this to the observations that both patients and carers talked more when using Talking Mats.

Case study 3: Ms A

(See the start of Ms A's case study in Chapter 3)

Ms A previously enjoyed craft and decoupage but has been reluctant to participate in this any more. She was recently diagnosed with primary progressive aphasia of the semantic variant after her family requested specialist assessment at a local memory clinic. Ms A has also been diagnosed with depression. Ms A presents with severe naming difficulties, single word comprehension and severely impaired writing skills on assessment using the BDAE. She expresses much frustration about these changes and now prefers to talk in a whisper, as she feels this doesn't highlight her word errors as much. One of her main concerns is that she is now unable to sign her name. Ms A reports that she used to be able to sign her craft works, and that if she could perhaps she would return to decoupage. One of the focuses of therapy was on introducing a writing task where Ms A was asked to study her written name, copy it and study it again. She was then encouraged to cover the previous examples and write it herself. She was asked to practise this at home, which she required significant encouragement to do. Ms A was eventually able to use a cover and copy system to write her name. She still required encouragement and set-up of equipment, but was able to work on some craft tasks and sign them using this technique.

In summary

At the beginning of this chapter, we highlighted that much of the work that we as clinicians can do with progressive language difficulties reflects the work we would ordinarily do with aphasic patients. And the limited evidence that there is in this area supports the effectiveness of this type of rehabilitation approach. There are simply a couple of additional variables to consider with these clients, the most relevant one being that this is a disease that is still going to progress, even whilst you are working on therapy. The research that has been done with patients with progressive language difficulties, particularly naming difficulties, demonstrates that impairment-based therapy can indeed maintain, if not improve, aspects of communication for some individuals. However, there is much to be done in developing language therapies for patients with dementia.

References

Bier, N., Macoir, J., Gagnon, L., Van der Linden, M., Louveaux, S,. & Desrosiers, J. (2009) Known, lost, and recovered: Efficacy of formal-semantic therapy and spaced retrieval method in a case of semantic dementia. *Aphasiology* **23**(2), 210–235.

Blackstone, S. & Hunt-Berg, M. (2012) *Social Networks: A Communication Inventory for Individuals with Complex Needs and their Partners. Revised version.* Attainment Company.

Bourgeois, M.S. & Hickey, E.M. (2009) *Dementia: From Diagnosis to Management – A Functional Approach*. New York: Psychology Press.

Cartwright, J. & Elliott, K.A.E. (2009) Promoting strategic television viewing in the context of progressive language impairment. *Aphasiology* **23**(2), 266–285.

Cherney, L.R., Halper, A.S., Holland, A., & Cole, R. (2008) Computerised script training for aphasia: Preliminary results. *American Journal of Speech Language Pathology* **17**, 19–34.

Croot, K. (2009) Progressive language impairments: Definitions, diagnoses, and prognoses. *Aphasiology* **23**(2), 302–326.

Croot, K., Nickels, L., Laurence, F., & Manning, M. (2009) Impairment- and activity/participation-directed interventions in progressive language impairment: Clinical and theoretical issues. *Aphasiology* **23**(2), 125–160.

Farrajota, L., Maruta, C., Maroco, J., Martins, I.P., Guerreiro, M., & De Mendonca, A. (2012) Speech therapy in primary progressive aphasia: A pilot study. *Dementia and Geriatric Cognitive Disorders Extra* **2**, 321–331.

Graham, K.S., Pratt, K.H., & Hodges, J.R. (1998) A reverse temporal gradient for public events in a single case of semantic dementia. *Neurocase: The Neural Basis of Cognition* **4**(6), 461–470.

Henry, M.L., Meese, M.V., Truong, S., Babiak, M., Miller, B.L., & Gorno-Tempini, M.L. (2012) Treatment for apraxia of speech in nonfluent variant primary progressive aphasia. *Behavioural Neurology* **25**, 1–10.

Heredia, C.G., Sage, K., Sage, M.A.L., & Berthier, M.L. (2009) Relearning and retention of verbal labels in a case of semantic dementia. *Aphasiology* **23**(2), 192–209.

Holland, A. (2008) Semantic memory and language processing in aphasia and dementia. Foreword. *Seminars in Speech and Language* **29**(1), 1.

Jokel, R., Rochon, E.A., & Leonard, C. (2006) Treatment for anomia in semantic dementia: Improvement, maintenance or both? *Neuropsychological Rehabilitation* **16**, 241–256.

Jokel, R., Cupit, J., Rochon, E., & Leonard, C. (2009) Relearning lost vocabulary in nonfluent progressive aphasia with MossTalk Words. *Aphasiology* **23**(2), 175–191.

Mayberry, E.J., Sage, K., Ehsan, S., & Ralph, M.A.L. (2011) Relearning in semantic dementia reflects contributions from both medial temporal lobe episodic and degraded neocortical semantic systems: Evidence in support of the complementary learning systems theory. *Neuropsychologia* **49**, 3591–3598

Murphy, J., Gray, C.M., & Cox, S. (2007) How 'Talking Mats' can help people with dementia to express themselves: Full report. Joseph Rowntree Foundation. Downloaded from: http://www.jrf.org.uk/sites/files/jrf/2128-talking-mats-dementia.pdf

Murphy, J., Oliver, T.M., & Cox, S. (2010) Talking Mats and involvement in decision making for people with dementia and family carers: Full Report. Joseph Rowntree Foundation. Downloaded from: http://www.jrf.org.uk/sites/files/jrf/Talking-Mats-and-decision-making-full.pdf

Murray, L.L. (1998) Longitudinal treatment of primary progressive aphasia: A case study. *Aphasiology* **12**(7), 651–672.

Papp, K.V., Walsh, S.J., & Snyder, P.J. (2009) Immediate and delayed effects of cognitive interventions in healthy elderly: A review of current literature and future directions. *Alzheimer's Dementia* **5**(1), 50–60.

Schneider, S.L., Thompson, C.K., & Luring, B. (1996) Effects of verbal plus gestural matrix training on sentence production in a patient with primary progressive aphasia. *Aphasiology* **10**(3), 297–317.

Speech and Language Therapy Psychiatry of Old Age Special Interest Group, November 2012, London.

Youmans, G., Holland, A., Munoz, M., & Bourgeois, M. (2005) Script training and automaticity in two individuals with aphasia. *Aphasiology* **19**(3–5), 435–450.

5 Therapy and management: Cognitive communication difficulties

Introduction

Cognitive difficulties are sometimes considered to be the domain of our neuropsychology colleagues. However, when they impact upon communication they may overlap into the domain of the speech and language therapist. Neuropsychologists' and speech and language therapists' skill sets complement one another in assessing and managing cognitive communication difficulties (Constantinidou et al., 2012). Indeed, both ASHA and the RCSLT state that speech and language therapists play a vital role in assessing and managing cognitive communication difficulties in people with dementia. ASHA even goes on to state that speech and language therapists are "the only professionals who are certified and licensed to treat communication disorders associated with cognitive deficits".

The previous chapter focused very specifically upon maintaining and improving the language of people living with progressive communication difficulties, with particular attention given to single words, sentences and reading and writing. In contrast, this chapter describes a series of individual and group-based interventions that have been shown to improve and maintain a variety of cognitive communication skills, including language, memory and various cognitive areas such as executive skills (verbal planning, attention, self-monitoring, awareness and judgement). Therapy approaches described here may also support more general aspects of communication such as mood and confidence.

Cognitive interventions can be categorized into three approaches (Papp, Walsh & Snyder, 2009; Claire, 2004) that comprise:

1. *Cognitive rehabilitation*: designed to improve performance on a specific task, an individualized approach where personally relevant goals are identified and the therapist works with the person and his or her family to devise strategies to address them.
2. *Cognitive training*: enhances specific cognitive skills through guided practice on a set of standard tasks such as paper-and-pencil or computer exercises
3. *Cognitive stimulation*: focuses on enhancing cognitive and social functioning through engagement in a range of activities and discussions (a group).

The challenge in planning therapy for patients with dementia, however, is not just about choosing and developing an intervention targeting current areas of difficulty. It is also around identifying a method that will maintain gains made even though therapy must be discontinued at some point, with the additional consideration of inevitable continued cognitive decline. Papp et al. (2009) highlight that there remains limited research in this area of intervention, and often the data and research have not kept up with the popularity of approaches being used in clinical practice. Consequently, it is all the more important that clinicians become aware of what evidence there is available and what limitations there may be in choosing certain therapy approaches.

The following chapter discusses both individual and group-based interventions in this area, and highlights the evidence currently available to underpin these approaches. As before, we also describe relevant case studies to support our discussion.

Individual therapy

Planning therapy for people with cognitive communication difficulties in dementia may require some creative thinking. Indeed, it is not uncommon that these clients have difficulties with motivation or may have limited learning abilities, even in the early stage of their disease (Bourgeois & Hickey, 2009). As the disease progresses, it may become even more challenging to establish any method of meaningful communication. Consequently, formal impairment-based tasks on their own may not be all that appropriate. This means therapy will need to be a little more dynamic, perhaps focusing on more functional strategies to support communication in a specific task. Finding ways to maintain a person's interest and maximize the impact of your approach could also include a combination of individual and group work. Group work will be discussed more in the next section but is an area where a number of different interventions have been developed and described in the literature.

Similarly to language-based interventions, the type of research available to support these cognitive communication therapies is limited, often based in expert opinion and case studies. But there have been some attempts to strengthen the evidence base for some of the better-established approaches such as validation therapy or intensive interaction. Table 5.1 provides an outline of some tasks and ideas for individual cognitive communication therapy.

Table 5.1 Therapy ideas for cognitive communication individual therapy.

Level of impairment	Suggested therapy tasks
Reduced pragmatics and self monitoring	Improving self monitoring: through education, video feedback and role play
Repetitious conversation/questions, poor topic maintenance, difficulties in conversing with people	External memory or communication aids: signage around home, review of diary or calendar management, memory/communication books, etc
Significantly disorientated to here and now (and somewhat agitated), little memory or recall	Validation therapy (see Group therapies)
Profoundly impaired: predominantly non-verbal or non-meaningful with repetitive behaviours that may be causing concern to staff and family	Intensive interaction/adaptive interaction SIMS apc (see SONAS apc under Group therapies)

Improving self-monitoring during conversation

During the milder stage of dementia some patients might already have developed subtle difficulties in conversation that they may not even realize, yet people around them are acutely conscious of. Some of these difficulties may include reduced awareness of social pragmatic rules including turn taking, topic maintenance, eye contact, body language and other often non-verbal conversational skills. Heightening an individual's awareness of a certain area of difficulty can aid them in monitoring it themselves without the need for constant external prompting and reducing the risk of conversational breakdown.

This can be done in just the same way as with an individual living with a non-progressive brain injury, be it stroke or traumatic brain injury, and include the use of questionnaires (Constantinidou et al., 2012) and reviewing video recordings of social interactions (Anderson, Anzalone, Holland & Tracey, 2011; Cornis-Pop, Mashima, Roth et al., 2012).

Many researchers have explored this therapy approach, particularly with people with aphasia such as Kagan and colleagues' work on Supported Conversation for Adults with Aphasia (Kagan, Black, Duchan, et al., 2001), and Lock, Wilkinson and Bryan's (2008) work on Supporting Partners of People with Aphasia in Relationships and Conversation (SPPARC). Both these approaches involve making a video of the person with communication difficulties having a conversation with their partner. After this, they are given some information about conversational rules such as turn taking, topic maintenance, and so on. Using the video clip to highlight where conversation is breaking down can support patients and their partners in identifying areas of strength and difficulty themselves, so enhancing their self-awareness outside of therapy sessions. This can also support patients to identify strategies together with the clinician and set goals that they feel more empowered to achieve. However, when planning this type of therapy with a patient with dementia a clinician must decide very carefully if the individual has retained enough awareness and memory to be able to apply this type of internal monitoring.

The concept of videoing a dyad and reviewing it together to identify areas for change and strategies that do or don't work well, overlaps with some of the work that might be done with conversation partners. Sometimes the unimpaired partner can benefit more than the person with dementia, who may find it difficult to take on strategies and apply them in lots of different situations. However, as previously mentioned, there will be more of a focus on conversation partners in Chapter 6.

What does the evidence say?

There are no examples of research specifically examining the use of video feedback to enhance communication skills for people with dementia. However, there are a couple of case studies that mention the use of this type of approach in their overview of the different things were trialled. These two examples are relatively dated now, but are still useful reference points in view of the paucity of literature on this topic. (See Chapter 6 for a further discussion on how this approach was integrated to carer training.)

Wong, Anand, Chapman et al. (2009) describes a case study named 'Bobby V'. The authors worked with Bobby V to develop his awareness of turn taking during the beginning stages of his PPA disease process. They tackled this by verbally educating Bobby V about the importance of turn taking in conversation. He was also invited to practise this in individual therapy sessions with his therapist by monitoring her non-verbal cues such as nodding her head and aiming to relinquish his turn when he observed these. He was interrupted if he did not pick up on them, and advised that he had missed a non-verbal cue. This was then practised in a group setting with his peers. Unfortunately, Wong et al. report little success with this technique.

Murray (1998) describes a case study named 'DD'. The author describes individual therapy sessions where she worked on DD's awareness of conversational breakdown. Murray describes how she explained to both DD and her spouse the turn taking and repair strategies they were using (based on pre-treatment conversational samples). They then discussed the effectiveness of their strategies as well as possible alternatives. Murray also staged role-play sessions with DD modelling target alternatives, which were videotaped. These were later examined and discussed by DD, her spouse and the author. This was combined with conversation partner training for DD's spouse. Following this intervention DD demonstrated improved or maintained performance on communication measures including the Communication Activities of Daily Living test (CADL) and the Communication Effectiveness Index (CETI; Lomas, Pickard, Bester, et al., 1989) and high ratings on the ASHA FACS.

External memory aids

As we all know, it is not uncommon that patients with dementia forget information. This can impact on the content of a conversation, the person's confidence in communication and the way they behave in a conversation. Communication difficulties in this situation can range from repetitive conversations, avoidance of communication situations, to difficulties in talking and being with loved ones. Bourgeois et al. (2009) explain that when people with memory loss associated with dementia experience a loss of memory that interrupts their train of thought, they will often switch to another topic and forget the earlier topic such that the conversation can break down. Patients may start to become distressed by their inability to participate in what they perceive as simple conversation. Family members and even carers will frequently describe frustration at having to repeat the same answer to the same question over and over again. Using external memory aids in these cases can assist in managing this concern and can act as a method of maintaining someone's independence, even in a conversation.

Bourgeois et al. (2009) explain that external strategies support retrieval of information from long-term memory storage through the environmental triggers they provide. This can take the form of strategically placed notes, signs and calendars. If patients can use these types of aids, it may reduce repetitive questions about daily routines or appointments, or prompt people to write a message after answering the telephone. For other patients, a personal memory or communication book may be helpful. Memory and communication books are certainly an area that speech and language therapists are familiar with. In this case, the therapist discusses with the patient and their loved ones what would be important to include, collecting photos and memorabilia, and developing a book of information to support memory and conversation. This may take the form of a small wallet for medical information, or family names and pictures or a detailed personal history memory book with written sentences and a picture to aid recall of particular events. This document can then support a person in conversation with other people, either by allowing them to refer to it for information, or by acting as another means of conveying information about themselves.

The thing I would stress, however, is the importance of training the patient (and their carers) to use these aids. Errorless learning and spaced retrieval is thought to be particularly useful when working with patients with Alzheimer's disease and vascular dementia who are relearning forgotten associations such as naming or sequences (Croot, Nickels, Laurence & Manning, 2009). However, errorless learning in this context can support the learning of a new sequence that includes a memory or communication aid. This is thought to work because it supports the learning of only correct items. Croot et al. (2009) cite Lambon, Ralph and Fillingham (2007) who explain that there are two learning systems, one that allows us to learn and strengthen specific associations (the Hebbian system), the other that allows us to monitor and correct our responses. It is thought that this second modulating system for learning is often impaired in these patients. This is similar to the theory of declarative and non-declarative memory described by Bourgeois et al. (2009), discussed in Chapter 4. Both theories suggest that by utilizing an errorless learning approach we reinforce specific associations between correct items and responses (utilizing the Hebbian system), and avoiding the learning of incorrect responses. This means that once a memory aid has been designed the patient will need to practise the sequence of events when the aid should be used, in the actual physical environment where the aid should be used. Using an errorless learning approach also means that you need to repeat the sequence whenever the patient fails to use the tool. For example, when repeatedly practising the use of the aid, the clinician will intervene immediately if an error is made and demonstrate the appropriate use, then allowing the patient to attempt the sequence again.

In embarking on this type of training it may be helpful to involve the people with whom the person with dementia communicates often, such as their carers and partners. In fact, by teaching carers and family members the errorless learning techniques they will be able to continue to reinforce this strategy outside of therapy sessions. This may simply require the person to prompt the person with dementia to use the memory aid, if they have failed to do so. For example, if the person asks repetitive questions about appointments, advise and refer them to the calendar. Other staff and family members may also benefit from education and training on how to use memory and communication books to support a conversation (this will be discussed in more detail in the next chapter).

What does the evidence say?

Evidence in this area of dementia and speech and language therapy is at best anecdotal, often focused on case studies. Perhaps this is because completing a randomized controlled trial in the use of memory and communication aids is difficult and challenging to say the least. But there are some descriptions in the literature that can guide our practice and reflection.

Bourgeois (2007) has published a manual describing the types and formats of different communication aids that can be used with this client group. Bourgeois et al. (2009) briefly describe this manual and also summarize a number of studies that the authors themselves have done examining the use of communication books in conversation between patients with dementia and their caregivers. They describe reduced repetitiveness, increased information exchange and reduced ambiguity in conversations. They also report increased balance in turn taking and topic maintenance as well as reduced need for partner prompting when memory aids were used. Perhaps one of the most useful for residential settings was the finding of enhanced cooperation and reduced problem behaviours when communication aids or memory books were used with care routines. In summarizing these studies they also highlight some of the limitations, particularly the cost and time required to train so many staff members in these specific approaches.

Case study 1: Mrs D

Mrs D is a 71-year-old lady who has just recently been diagnosed with vascular dementia. She lives with her daughter in a two-bedroom house. One of the things she and her daughter notice most is that she frequently forgets her appointments, both social events and medical appointments. This has started to have an impact on her health, as she has missed some important blood tests. She has also started to feel low and attributes this to the fact that she has missed her social group meeting a number of times recently. Mrs D and her daughter have started arguing frequently and her daughter reported feeling frustrated by her mother at times. Mrs D's daughter goes to work a few hours every day and is not able to be there to prompt her mother all the time. In fact, she is becoming increasingly frustrated and concerned that she won't be able to continue going to work. Both Mrs D and her daughter feel they are quite good at writing things down; each have their own diary and a couple of calendars and they use Post-it notes. On closer questioning, Mrs D revealed that appointments don't always make it from a Post-it note to the calendar. In fact, they seem to be kept in two or three different places around the kitchen. Furthermore, each calendar and diary has different information in it, which doesn't always correspond. Working alongside the occupational therapist, the speech and language therapist was able to identify one calendar, which both Mrs D and her daughter share and which they pin to the fridge. They agreed that, from now on, all appointments will be pinned to the fridge and transferred to one calendar. Every Sunday night, Mrs D's daughter checks the forthcoming week, and Mrs D documents these on the calendar using an agreed format: red for medical appointments and black for all other items. If Mrs D starts questioning her daughter about appointments her daughter directs her to the calendar rather than checking everything for her. In order to ensure this system works they need to practise at home repeatedly with the therapists, using an errorless approach. They also practise together when the therapists are not present. As a result, they both feel more on top of their appointments and, even if problems arise, they are able to problem solve together using their 'memory corner' on the fridge. Mrs D's daughter continues to go to work and feels less concerned about her mother's memory. They also report fewer arguments in day-to-day conversations.

Adaptive interaction/Intensive interaction

Intensive interaction therapy was first developed in the 1980s for people with severe learning difficulties. More recently, it has been used to support people with profound dementia. The main premise of intensive interaction therapy is that all behaviour is viewed as intentional communication. This means that any non-verbal behaviours are considered as meaningful as any intentional communication acts. An example of this could be that of a patient chewing their fingers or repeatedly banging their fist on the side of their bed. These types of behaviours in particular could cause people around the patient to become concerned about their wellbeing. But any behaviour will be interpreted as conveying some type of communication.

By the time dementia reaches the later stages patients may seem 'completely unreachable', and consequently carers will generally no longer attempt to engage them in social interactions. Care staff and families may simply continue interactions solely to complete basic daily care activities. Ellis and Estell (2008) advocate that these patients still demonstrate some urge and ability to communicate through their 'behaviours'. And, ultimately, intensive interaction aims to engage patients with dementia in meaningful communication interactions with the people working with them.

One might say that intensive interaction therapy focuses on 'the moment'. During the therapy sessions the main focus is on the process of the interaction rather than any specific outcome. The principles of the interactions are considered to reflect the type of communication that happens in early infant life between caregivers and infants and which are primarily non-verbal. This process requires the clinician to get to know the patient and then engage in a type of reflective behaviour, for example mirroring some things the patient does, or redirecting the person to develop the repertoire of interactions. The focus is generally on turn taking, shared attention and eye gaze. This is achieved through shared body language, eye gaze, vocalizations and facial expressions that are meaningful to the person with dementia. Some clinicians may choose to introduce simple objects to this process; this is not always considered a 'pure' intensive interaction approach but this is a broad debate. Caldwell (2005, cited by Ellis & Astell, 2008) explains that for the learning disabled this intensive interaction develops to a shared language. The aim is then that, over time, therapy sessions direct individuals from solitary behaviours, such as biting, to meaningful shared activity.

What does the evidence say?

As with communication interventions described previously, there are almost no examples of robust 'research' into the use of this technique with people with dementia. But there is one published case study by Ellis et al. (2008). They describe a case where they used intensive interaction with an almost non-verbal patient who had a diagnosis of dementia. Ellis et al. (2008) emphasize that, when communicating with clients with dementia, one should not make an assumption that a common repertoire can be built up over a series of interactions due to the clients' likely severe memory problems. They suggest each interaction must be approached as a unique encounter where the clinician must adapt their communication anew. They therefore renamed the approach 'adaptive interaction'.

Ellis et al.'s (2008) case study 'Edie' lives in a care home and is generally immobile. They started by observing her and liaising with staff and family about her communication. It was felt by those interviewed that Edie's behaviours, such as thumb chewing, high-pitched sounds and laughing, held some intention. Consequently, they compared her communication across two sessions: one focused on asking her questions and awaiting responses, the other was an 'adaptive interaction' session. They found that in verbal conversation Edie quickly disengaged, whilst in intensive interaction she continued to participate in turn taking for a much longer period. They also found that when the clinician mirrored Edie's communication, in particular her eye contact and high-pitched sounds, this led to Edie introducing movement and touch. In comparison, when participating in verbal conversation she closed her eyes and became very still, indicating disengagement. Ellis et al. (2008) suggest that this type of therapy may be a potential 'tool for promoting and supporting communication between people with advanced dementia and those who care for them' and advocate for further research and debate in the literature on this topic. There is further research currently in development in this promising therapeutic area for people with dementia (Harris, unpublished). This will contribute to the literature and support the clinical application of intensive interaction.

Case study 2: Mr E

Mr E was a 71-year-old Irish gentleman with Alzheimer's dementia who had been living in a residential facility for around four years. Mr E had been mobile and verbal when he first came to the nursing home and staff

> described him as a respectful man who showed much fondness for staff. He previously enjoyed listening to classical music and walking in the garden with his wife. His dementia had progressed and he now stayed in bed and was totally dependent on others, being physically passive with a tense and contracted body tone. He no longer used any verbal language, but spent much of his waking hours vocalising loudly, often with his eyes closed. The tone of his vocalisations suggested that he may have been agitated or bored. The speech and language therapist followed the positive response schedule (PRS) described by Perrin (1997). During intensive interaction sessions Mr E continued to vocalise but the tone was very different. Gradually it began to sound more like the speech and language therapist's vocalisations, and there was more variety in his intonation. He seemed calmer and more responsive. Mr E started to make a number of deliberate head and body movements during sessions, in response to the speech and language therapist, initiating touch and responding to the tapping of a beat on his thumb. He made extensive eye contact and would occasionally move the therapist's hand to another position. After the course of intervention finished staff commented that Mr E had become more responsive, opening his eyes more and looking at them when they called his name. (From Harris, unpublished with copyright permission)

Group therapy

Speech and language therapists looking for ideas and research about what group therapy approaches may be effective when working with people with dementia will find that there is actually a significant amount of information. From this plethora of information, it is obvious that reminiscence therapy and cognitive stimulation therapy are some of the most researched and perhaps most commonly-used approaches. Yet most clinicians would agree that education groups have their place for some of the more mildly impaired patients. It is also noteworthy that some approaches, such as reality orientation, have become quite outdated for use with people with dementia. Other newer approaches, such as intensive interaction and Sonas apc, are instead becoming more commonplace in clinical practice.

Running a group, however, is not always as straightforward as it sounds, and I would encourage clinicians to consider attending group facilitation training at some point in their early work life. Not only do you need to think carefully about whom you will be including in your groups, but about how exactly you will run the group, where and how long you will run it for and how you will measure its effectiveness. Facilitating a group of communication-impaired adults requires much skill and attention to ensure the participation of each member, use of appropriate cueing, limiting inappropriate conversation but encouraging the development of the 'group milieu' – a most valuable therapeutic tool.

The following provides a discussion of some of these group therapy approaches and directs you to the evidence that supports their rationale. This will equip you with the basis of the information; but keeping abreast of changes in this area of practice is valuable. It is easier to keep up-to-date with some of the more widely-researched group therapy approaches as free sources of information such as the Cochrane Library have published reviews of, for example, cognitive stimulation therapy. In fact, national guidelines and policies are also able to support these therapies as evidence for them becomes more robust. Table 5.2 provides a summary of therapy ideas for cognitive communication group sessions.

Table 5.2 Therapy ideas for cognitive communication group sessions.

Level of impairment	Suggested therapy tasks
Mildly impaired: anxious to understand what implications their condition may have, mobile and independent in most aspects of daily life (perhaps living with a partner or family member who helps in daily activities)	Education groups Cognitive stimulation therapy Combined exercise and communication groups
More moderately impaired but still able to actively engage in a more traditional group setting	Reality orientation Cognitive stimulation therapy Reminiscence groups Validation therapy SONAS apc groups Combined exercise and communication groups
Moderate–severely impaired patients with dementia living in residential type settings (who may struggle to engage in verbal conversation)	SONAS apc groups

Education groups

Empowerment is a concept described by the World Health Organization as a 'prerequisite for health' which improves health outcomes and quality of life among the chronically ill (Segolene, Kole & Groft, 2008). Empowerment of patients can lead to improvements in individual effective decision-making, problem solving, management of disease complications and improved health behaviours. In other words, intervention for people living with dementia shouldn't always just focus on maximizing and improving functions. Supporting people to feel confident in coping with their condition and helping them develop their own strategies to reduce stress and manage in daily life can be just as effective as traditional therapy (Kasl-Godley & Gatz, 2000).

Education groups are frequently the first type of group someone with dementia may be invited to. And although these types of groups are still not routinely part of a speech and language therapy service, they are often run by charity organizations such as the Frontotemporal Dementia Support Group or the Alzheimer's Association. Yet it is increasingly recognized that this type of group can improve patients' ability to self-manage for longer without requiring such regular therapy input.

In my experience, education groups that have been run by clinicians are often run by a number of clinicians together, with a therapist or nurse specialist acting to facilitate the session and ensure information is presented in a format to suit each participant's communication needs. Education and self-efficacy groups are frequently also described as support or psycho-education groups and may be co-facilitated by a psychologist. Whatever the case, these types of groups can form part of rehabilitation for cognitive and communication difficulties for people with dementia.

Education and self-efficacy groups focus on teaching people with dementia (and their partners) compensatory strategies within the group sessions, setting practical exercises and practising these either within the group or as home assignments. Participants are then able to spend some time sharing their concerns, and problem-solving difficulties along the way. Ideally, facilitators of these types of client-centered groups seek information from patients, prior to the sessions even starting, about what they would like to achieve by attending the groups, and then use these goals as a guide to ensure sessions are relevant and useful. This often includes planning the group 'curriculum' in the first session with patients present, planning individual session themes and inviting other professionals to present on particular subjects (see Table 5.3 for an example of a group curriculum).

Table 5.3 Example of an overview of what an education/self efficacy group might include (taken from Cahill, Busssolaro, Volkmer & Hopkins, 2010).

OT = occupational therapist; SP = speech pathologist

Week	Facilitator	Session overview
1	OT/SP/Medical	Introduction, goals overview, sharing personal experiences. Medical overview of cognitive changes
2	OT/SP	Cognitive strategies: External and internal
3	OT/SP	Using strategies in everyday life
4	SP/OT	Communication management
5	SP/OT/Social Work	Listening to your partners
6	SP/OT/Social Work	Accessing community resources
7	OT/SP/Nursing	Lifestyle management
8	OT/SP	Conclusion: Future planning and client goal review

What does the evidence say?

The evidence for education groups and self-efficacy for patients with dementia is relatively tricky to examine, as different professional groups often publish it under a variety of different titles. It is also an area where the best examples are often from shared best practice rather than robust research trials. However, the evidence is generally positive, if vague and non-specific. Indeed, few articles explain the programme content in great specificity, nor are group formats in general explained. And, frequently, it appears that different patients groups may be mixed together which, although more clinically realistic, makes it trickier to examine and pick apart specific outcomes for different client groups.

At any rate, the NICE guidelines for dementia (NICE, 2011) do include an entire section on training and education for people with dementia, their carers and staff. In this section, they report that there is not a strong evidence base around educating patients with dementia, attributing this to the fact that this is a fairly 'young' area in terms of research. Yet they emphasize the value of these programmes as people are increasingly being viewed as 'expert patients', who are important members of the team in managing their own conditions. The guideline does describe two studies examining the value of general dementia education programmes (Zaret et al., 2004 and Bird et al., 2004, cited in NICE, 2011). These studies highlight that participants report significant enjoyment in attending these types of education and support groups.

The literature on cognitive impairment is generally providing increasingly positive data demonstrating the value of education groups. Indeed, clients with cognitive disorders have reported improvements in memory-related self-efficacy and reduced anxiety after attending a series of group education sessions (Metternich, Schmidke, Dykierek & Hull, 2008; Troyer, Murphy, Anderson, Moscovitch & Craik, 2008). Multidisciplinary memory programmes have also resulted in participants using more strategies, with gains maintained three months later (Troyer et al., 2008). Other researchers have shown that groups can have a positive impact on acceptance of disease or impairment and potentially improve marital satisfaction (Joosten-Weyn Bannigh, Kessels, Rikkert, Geleijins-Lanting & Kraaimaat, 2008). Indeed, more recently, Cahill et al. (2010) were able to demonstrate that using goal setting measures to guide group planning in a self-management group specifically for people with dementia led to reduced perception of carer burden and increased participant confidence.

Looking through the progressive aphasia literature, some of the case studies also reference attendance at aphasia groups. These are not always progressive groups but may include a mixture of clients including non-progressive aphasics (Murray, 1998). These types of case studies and examples are perhaps where we can glean some excellent examples of good clinical practice. Even if the evidence is not in randomized controlled trial format, it is valuable advice and guidance to what to include if you are considering this type of group in your service: i.e. being patient-centered in topic choice, focusing on practical assignments and problem solving within each session and, finally, encouraging people to feel more confident in their own skills. Developing self-efficacy is a whole topic unto itself and there is much information on this in other parts of the literature. I would strongly advise that any clinician planning an education and self-efficacy group should read up on this approach to enhance their skills in this area.

Case study 3: Mr F

Mr F was invited to attend a communication education group with his wife. He had just been diagnosed with vascular dementia about six months before. He and his wife lived locally in a warden-controlled flat. His wife identified that they were having difficulties managing his condition, which regularly resulted in arguments. Mr F felt that his word-finding and memory difficulties contributed, but that he wasn't sure how to manage this at times and his wife and family didn't really understand this aspect of his condition. They felt they needed some advice on communicating with one another and on how his family could productively support him. A speech and language therapist and an occupational therapist jointly facilitated the group sessions. Topics were chosen to ensure they addressed Mr F's concern (as well as concerns voiced by other members of the group). This meant that the facilitators spent some time providing brain education and explaining how language and cognition can be affected. They also provided written information, such as the Alzheimer's Society information sheets, for participants to take away and give to other family members. Other sessions focused on communication and memory strategies, and problem solving when conversation broke down and reminders failed. This included group discussion and use of vignettes. Finally, a guest speaker was invited to attend the group to discuss the adjustment process to living with dementia (led by a social worker). Mr F and his wife did bring up their concerns in the group, and were surprised and relieved when others described similar feelings. Mr and Mrs F were able to trial the use of strategies between sessions and returned to discuss their limitations and successes at later group sessions. Mr and Mrs F reported that they felt their concerns had been addressed by the group but that they would be actively seeking further speech and language therapy input should things change with Mr F's communication in the future. They also professed they had not been aware of this service prior to attending the group sessions. They became close friends with another couple in the group, and started seeing them socially which they reported as a great source of support.

Cognitive stimulation therapy

Cognitive stimulation can be traced to the USA in the 1950s when it was initially associated with reality orientation. The purpose of reality orientation was to maintain skills by providing prompts and cues through a set of orientation facts, e.g. the date, location and weather today. This was discussed in a group, one-to-one conversation with carers, or a combination of both. This approach was considered quite a rigid and confrontational approach, where 'classes' were held once or twice daily for 30 minutes. Basic personal and current information was presented and a reality orientation board was used to list the unit, location, day, date, weather, etc.

Since the 1990s, reality orientation has been practised much less due to its inflexible structure and lack of meaningful impact, as well as the risk of possible negative effects on individuals' wellbeing. More recently, some aspects of this programme have been modified to form cognitive stimulation. Cognitive stimulation was designed as a three-part cognitive remediation programme including memory, problem solving and conversation activities delivered by a trained caregiver and using an instruction workbook of graded activities. These activities focus on word fluency, verbal recall, verbal recognition, problem solving, planning and categorization. Some researchers describe sessions being held six days per week, for one hour per day for up to 12 weeks. In a clinical setting, this is more likely to be one day per week, for up to an hour, over an 8–12-week period. Sessions will often follow a format whereby a group song is sung, patients discuss the day, date, season and other orientation information using a paper and signage to support the conversation. Patients participate in two activities such as looking at photos, maps and papers and discuss these, completing word play tasks listed above, sharing and discussing foods and flavours or some such stimulation task (according to the theme of the week) before finishing with the group song. Spector, Thorgrimsen, Woods et al. (2006) wrote a week-by-week guide for cognitive stimulation therapy, which was more recently updated by Aguirre, Spector, Streater et al. (2011).

National and international organizations have made recommendations about the use of cognitive stimulation therapy with patients with dementia. Indeed, the NICE SCEI guidelines (2011) recommend that all people with mild-to-moderate dementia should have the opportunity to participate in cognitive stimulation groups. The 2011 World Alzheimer's report (Prince, Bryce, & Ferri, 2011) states that "we found strong evidence (multiple RCTS) that cognitive stimulation (for cognitive function) is an effective intervention in mild dementia". And they state that, consequently, "these interventions should therefore be routinely offered" to people with mild Alzheimer's disease.

What does the evidence say?

Since reality orientation is no longer such a commonly-used approach, because of its potential negative effects on wellbeing, it is not really worthwhile to evaluate much of the research in this area. Suffice to say that Bourgeois et al. (2009) summarize some of the evidence for reality orientation and highlight that reality orientation has produced increased scores on measures of verbal orientation compared to no treatment. This has resulted in many nursing homes, wards and residential facilities adopting the use of a board which provides this information somewhere on the ward. Unfortunately these are often poorly situated and staff do not necessarily use them systematically with patients. Bourgeois et al. (2009) highlight that individuals may be better equipped with individualized memory wallet or cue cards with more specific, personally relevant information on them.

As mentioned previously, when compared to other therapy approaches for communication in dementia there is a relative plethora of evidence supporting the use of cognitive stimulation therapy. In fact, cognitive stimulation therapy is perhaps one of the few areas of therapy for people with dementia where there have been a reasonable number of randomized controlled trials. Many of these research articles have even been reviewed in a Cochrane report (most recently in 2012). This is one of the most helpful documents you can read about this therapy approach and is very easily accessible (for free) via the Cochrane Library website. There is little to say here, but that: "There is evidence from a (small) number of studies that cognitive stimulation may be associated with improvements in quality of life and communication" (Woods, Aguirre, Spector & Orrell, 2012)

The following provides a summary of the content of the Cochrane review and a number of studies included in this review on the topic of cognitive stimulation therapy.

The most recent Cochrane review on the topic of cognitive stimulation therapy (Woods et al., 2012) considered only randomized controlled trials for which there was adequate information in English. These trials all had to be published in a peer-reviewed journal and meet the definition of cognitive stimulation therapy described by Claire (2004). Finally, participants were required to attend for a minimum of four weeks according to the inclusion criteria for the review. Woods et al. (2012) included 13 studies in their review. Participants were over 70 years on average and from all different settings including care homes, outpatient and hospital in-patient settings. The median session length was 45 minutes (with a range of 30–90 minutes), median session frequency was three times per week (with a range of between one and five times per week). Group sizes varied from between five and seven, but also included one study where a family member provided the therapy following a training period. Tasks included reality orientation tasks such as using a reality orientation board, discussion of newspapers, photos, calenders and clocks to focus on orientation as well as drawing, word association/categorization and naming tasks, or discussion around the past, hobbies, activities, and dementia education. Some groups used the manual designed by Spector et al. (2006) to guide week-by-week session plans of topics and tasks. In comparison, the control groups for these trials all did very different activities ranging from nothing (treatment as usual) to watching TV, physiotherapy and a reminiscence group. The studies' outcomes included mini mental state examination (MMSE), the Alzheimer's disease assessment scale-cognitive (ADAS-cog), self-rating of quality of life and depression measures as well as carer and family rating scales. The communication scale most commonly used was the Holden Communication Scale.

There were a number of positive effects of cognitive stimulation therapy outlined in the Cochrane review. Results demonstrated that there is a positive impact on communication and social interaction even outside of the sessions, as well as improved quality of life. Spector and Orell (2010) also demonstrated that language function improved on direct testing following attendance at cognitive stimulation therapy. The largest effect were for groups where participants attended for longer than 12 months, and in a couple of studies the effects on cognitive function were shown to be maintained for a period of time after participants had stopped attending. These studies demonstrated maintenance at 3 months post therapy. There was no information on the cost-effectiveness of such an intervention in this review. However, a study by Knapp et al. (2006, cited in NICE, 2011) compared cognitive stimulation therapy to standard care for people with mild-to-moderate dementia. The objective of this study was to investigate the resource implications and cost-effectiveness of cognitive stimulation in care homes and day centres. The evidence indicated that, in the UK, providing cognitive stimulation therapy alongside usual care for people with mild-to- moderate dementia in both care homes and day-care centres is likely to be more cost effective than usual care alone

There were, however, a number of limitations to the studies highlighted by the Cochrane review. No trial managed to blind the assessors and participants to their treatment trial. In fact, there was even the risk of contamination between groups who were in close contact. It was equally difficult to blind all assessors to outcomes, particularly when completing staff ratings. Some trials did not provide detailed treatment protocols and although those facilitators who were not speech and language therapists were given training, it was still difficult to demonstrate how consistency of provision was monitored. There was generally a lack of clarity around randomization procedures in the studies. And often low numbers of people participated in the research. However, these factors are evidently being addressed with more recent studies which, for example, particularly focus on higher sample sizes. The authors of the review also emphasize that more research is required to highlight the impact of cognitive stimulation therapy on different dementia subtypes and the mild versus more moderately impaired groups.

However, the evidence has not yet demonstrated whether these results can be maintained beyond three months. This means that, when considering the use of cognitive stimulation therapy in a clinical setting, it is worth planning how you could support the maintenance of these effects – i.e. how you will continue to run the groups once they are set up. Will you train others, e.g. rehabilitation assistants, nursing staff or even more junior therapists? And how will you ensure the quality of this therapy is maintained, what kind of supervision, mentorship or regular review process will you employ? Spector, Thorgrimsen, Wood, et al. (2003) also highlight a major difference between the study participants and a real clinical situation, suggesting that exclusion criteria in these studies is often more rigorous than real clinical situations. This is important for clinicians to be aware of when inviting some participants to attend. Consider carefully if patients will benefit from this type of therapy, and whether they will be able to participate in the group appropriately rather than causing disruptions for others, for example.

Case study 4: Mrs G

Mrs G was admitted from a local nursing home to the acute older adult mental health ward due to the changes in her behaviour. She was a lady who had a history of Lewy body disease. She would spend her time moving from chair to chair around the ward and talking loudly with people who were not there (hallucinating). These were all people from her younger life, and about whom she would describe complex confabulations. Staff were finding her behaviour challenging as she would often become loud and irritably aggressive if she was interrupted. Staff attempted to orientate her to her surroundings and certain times of day, such as lunch times. Mrs G started to attend the cognitive stimulation group on the ward, with three other patients. The group ran once a week for an hour over an 8-week period. Most patients were admitted to the ward for at least three or four months so this generally meant they were able to engage in at least one entire cycle of the group sessions. Mrs G started attending the group regularly. The group format followed that written by Spector; this meant that each session included an introductory song (which was chosen by the group and sung every week). Some basic orientation to the ward, season and date was also included. One or two new activities were introduced every week that centered around word generation, reminiscence, discussion of topical subjects such as the Olympics, Christmas and the weather. Mrs G attended all these sessions without becoming irritated once. Through the course of the group we also found out her love of singing and her ability to engage in word play tasks. In the group, Mrs G was orientated to the tasks, she rarely engaged with her hallucinations and was easily able to be refocused to task when she did. Outside of session, staff were able to carry over her love of singing and would often use a spontaneous sing-along as a way to reduce any apparent agitation.

Reminiscence

Reminiscence therapy is the process of recalling episodes from one's past (Kim, Cleary, Hopper, et al., 2006). Some authors distinguish between reminiscence and life review by suggesting that reminiscence is the process of recalling the past whilst life review is the evaluation of those events. However, both reminiscence therapy and life review aim to facilitate recall of past experiences to promote intrapersonal and interpersonal functioning and thereby improve wellbeing (Kasl-Godley & Gatz, 2000). And it is generally agreed that reminiscence provides a structured way to interact with others in a group setting. Psychologically, reminiscence is associated with positive changes in self-esteem and increased life satisfaction. This is achieved through intrapersonal reflection, giving meaning to one's life and providing resolution. Whilst cognitively it is thought that reminiscence decreases demands on impaired cognitive abilities and capitalizes on preserved ones, because people with dementia are more likely to have preserved remote autobiographical memory so discussing previous life events will result in enhanced communicative interactions.

Reminiscence therapy normally uses props such as pictures and objects (often personally relevant scrapbooks/photo albums, etc). It may be conducted through individual one-to-one conversations using, for example, a memory book, via a multimedia computer-based reminiscence package (Alm, Astell, Ellis, et al, 2004) or in a group setting sharing stories with others. Speech and language therapists often use reminiscence to reduce social isolation by encouraging interactions between older adults and other communication partners (Kim et al., 2006). Speech and language therapists can be involved in assessing and screening processes to ensure that patients are appropriate candidates for this type of therapy, as well as assisting in the design and implementation of the therapy in the clinical setting.

What does the evidence tell us?

The research literature in this area is generally somewhat dated. Kasl-Godley and Gatz reviewed the evidence available for reminiscence therapy in 2000. Later, a systematic review of papers related to reminiscence therapy was conducted by a committee established by the Academy of Neurologic Communication Disorders and Sciences in collaboration with the American Speech-Language Hearing Association (Kim, Cleary, Hopper et al., 2006). This committee found six studies that were judged to provide class II level evidence to support the use of reminiscence therapy, including most of the articles described by Kasl-Godley et al. (2000). In general, these papers are quite dated (e.g. Goldwasser et al., 1987; Head et al., 1990, cited in ASHA, 2006). Yet all the papers demonstrated general improvements in patients' mood, staff knowledge of patients and therefore interactions with staff outside of the groups.

Kim et al. (2006) found that although most of the six studies compared the treatment groups to control groups, only one of these used a randomized process to assign patients. Kim et al. report that of the total 122 participants included in all these studies, individuals were rarely given a diagnosis more specific than dementia, and only one study included patients specifically with Alzheimer's disease, multi-infarct dementia and vascular dementia. Furthermore, and perhaps most importantly for us as clinicians, little information was given about the procedure for reminiscence sessions and only one study described a standardized protocol (Bruce, Hodgson & Schweitzer (1999) Reminiscing with People with Dementia: A Handbook for Carers).

Validation therapy

Validation therapy is a method of communicating with an individual in whatever time or location they think it is so their feelings are recognized and acknowledged. This is thought to improve emotional and social functioning by supporting patients in the process of coping with the cognitive, emotional, and social consequences of their condition (Burgio & Fisher, 2000). This approach is based on the concept that people with dementia progress through four stages of resolving personal conflict: mal-orientation, time confusion, repetitive motion and vegetation (Feil cited by Bourgeois & Hickey, 2009). Feil emphasizes the use of non-verbal communication –touch, eye contact, and tone of voice – to facilitate this process. This can take the form of reassuring touches on the arm, vocalizing positively to encourage people to continue speaking (for example, a simple 'aha') and sitting with the person, engaging in active listening or just being in each other's company. The aim of validation therapy is to treat behavioural symptoms such as disruptive vocalization and wandering. Validation therapy sessions are often performed in a group setting, but speech and language therapists frequently use aspects of validation in their individual interactions with patients to build trust and rapport during a session.

What does the evidence tell us?

There seems to be very little published research available that examines the effectiveness of validation therapy with people with dementia. What was available seemed to demonstrate little evidence of the positive effect of this approach compared to other therapies. In fact, it appears that there is little advantage to using validation therapy other than that staff might change their perspectives on patients.

Burgio and Fisher (2000) cite a study by Toseland and colleagues (1997) who compared a validation group to a normal social group. The researchers found that, after a year of therapy, group members were less aggressive within the social group, although they continued in their use of repetitive behaviours such as wandering, hiding objects and so on. In comparison, members of the social group demonstrated a decrease in these behaviours.

More recently, Bourgeois and Hickey (2009) reviewed the literature on validation therapy approaches and concluded that the evidence for validation therapy is mostly anecdotal. They reported that the evidence from these groups has been equivocal and focuses on improved mood and enjoyment but little generalization. Perhaps the most positive aspect is that the involvement of nursing staff has shown to change staff perceptions of residents (Gibson, 1994, cited in Bourgeois & Hickey, 2009). They did emphasize the value of this treatment as a technique for more advanced dementia but highlighted the need for further investigation.

Sensory stimulation

Sensory stimulation sessions have been often described in the literature (Burgio & Fisher, 2000) and generally incorporate music, physical activity, smell and touch. Sonas aPc differs from these groups in that it focuses on communication through sensory activities. Sister Mary Threadgold developed Sonas aPc (activating potential for communication) as a therapy approach in Dublin in 1990. These groups were designed specifically for people with dementia and cognitive communication impairments. The aim of these groups is to promote wellbeing through interaction, hence 'Sonas', which means wellbeing or contentment in Gaelic. The theory behind the Sonas approach is that it 'touches into each level above the biological needs' (Threadgold, 2002). Threadgold (2002) cites O'Connor and Seymour (1990) to help explain how this impacts on communication. They state, "If the loop of communication has any beginning, it starts with the senses." Indeed, through sight we understand things such as the time of year, someone's facial expression and are able to interpret their gestures. Through hearing we understand words, but also vocal tone and any environmental sounds. Through smell we become aware of someone's presence and perhaps where we are (for example, that we are in the kitchen where a meal is about to be served). Through touch we understand our interpersonal relationship and through taste we understand what food we are eating. Many behavioural problems, such as resistance to care and physical or verbal aggression, agitation and restlessness, can arise from sensory deprivation, unskillful caregiver–patient interactions and patients' fear and loneliness (Hamill & Connors, 2004). They highlight that improving communication can help build relationships and, consequently, participation in daily activities. Sonas aPc is an approach that attempts to maximize the communication environment of people with dementia in order for them to realize their communication potential (Hamill & Connorss, 2004). This means adjusting the environment to suit the patients' communication and sensory needs.

The Sonas aPc groups are designed as a multisensory packaged programme, using music, song, touch and smell to promote interaction. The sessions use a one-hour tape-recorded package that follows the same weekly format. Sessions include activities such as singing – both group signature songs and sing-alongs – massage, stimulation of smell and taste such as aromatherapy oils, gentle exercises, music and poetry and some memory-focused exercises. The repetitive structure provided by the tape recording is considered important in order to familiarize people with dementia to the programme. It also allows the clinician to focus more on the individuals attending (Brown, 1997). The aim of the group is to enhance participants' communication abilities rather than disabilities (Threadgold & Grennan, 2003; Threadgold, 2002). This approach was originally designed as a group therapy but has also been modified as an individual therapy called SIMS (sonas individual multisensory session). In order to practise this type of therapy, basic training can be completed through attendance at a two-day workshop.

People who attend and consequently deliver the sonas aPc 'package' do not necessarily need to have a professional qualification. Similarly to cognitive stimulation therapy it is often the rehabilitation assistants and nursing aides who conduct ongoing aPc sessions in the long term.

What does the evidence tell us?

Sonas aPc groups have been described anecdotally in clinical magazines and books but little formalized research has been conducted with this client group. The main outcomes described by both clinicians and the limited research available appear generally qualitative. And the research studies that have been done are now fairly dated.

Threadgold (1995, 2002) describes how Sonas can facilitate communication, increase awareness, encourage interaction, initiative and involvement, trigger memories and provide relaxation and enjoyment. They report that research undertaken by SONAS aPc TM has shown improvement in cognitive ability, reduction in behavioural problems and improved communication in activities of daily living. They report that, in 1996, Linehan and Birkbeck found a positive effect in most of these areas (unpublished work).

Connors (2000) was able to show more measurable improvements in these areas using the Mini Mental State Examination (MMSE), the Geriatric Depression

Rating scale, the Baumgarten Dementia Rating Scale, the Blessed-Roth scale and the Holden 5-point Communication scale. These positive outcomes were also demonstrated in a repeat study by the same authors in 2001. This study included a comparison to a control group, who demonstrated no significant changes in any domain. There are many limitations to the methodology of these studies, including no indication of whether improvements will be maintained without ongoing therapy.

Baker (2001) describes how she approached the implementation of Sonas aPc in her clinical practice, highlighting that patients actively choose to continue attending Sonas aPc groups. Baker also reflected that it has had an impact on other aspects of therapy she does, outside of the groups, including the type of information she incorporates into life-story-books. For example she now includes questions such as 'what was the person's favourite perfume' into her research when developing these books.

Black (2005) also describes conducting Sonas aPc groups together with her occupational therapy colleagues and observes that people who are unable to communicate with one another on the ward are able to converse within the sessions. She suggests that these groups allow patients to relax and give them the time and opportunity to communicate through a variety of modalities. Black does, however, highlight some of the limitations to using this therapy with people with dementia. She states: "It is impossible to argue how clinically effective this type of therapy is. Working with a client group regressing along a conclusively deteriorating pathway means one does not expect hugely positive steps."

This evidence, although methodologically weak, supports the use of Sonas aPc as a clinically useful intervention for people with dementia in a clinical setting. Unfortunately, it is likely that employing this type of approach would require significant financial and time investment. Not only are facilitators required to attend a special training course but will probably require regular support from a speech and language therapist in continuing to run groups (Hamill & Connors, 2004). It is also recommended that participants should continue to attend the Sonas aPc sessions indefinitely in order to maintain gains made (Threadgold, 2002).

Combined exercise and communication groups

Arkin and Mahendra (2001) and Mahendra and Arkin (2003) developed innovative treatment programmes for people with dementia in which they have combined multiple approaches – exercises, communication and social interaction tasks – into one treatment, using volunteers to support the programme. They have demonstrated improvements in people's communication skills through this balanced 'healthy living' approach.

Arkin and Mahendra (2001) describe a programme of therapy for a small group of Alzheimer's patients in which they measured the impact of physical and language interventions on discourse outcomes. They compared two groups where one was provided with a twice-weekly exercise regime and language intervention, whilst the other was provided with only a twice-weekly exercise programme. Both groups also received one session a week with a volunteer in the second semester focusing on social interaction and conversation. The language intervention focused on picture description tasks, fluency exercises, advice and opinion questions, naming and language games. They hypothesized that repeated activation of a concept in these exercises would strengthen the association between a stimulus and the retrieved information. The authors suggested this could trigger a chain reaction stimulating retrieval of other words and concepts (Arkin & Mahendra, 2001). They also observed that discussing topics other than food and care needs is validating, and noted that a previous study by Mueller (1993) has shown the positive effect of discussing moral issues on self esteem. Arkin and Mahendra found their programme demonstrated an improvement on noun use and mental status for the patients participating in both exercise and language intervention. However, the number of participants in the study was very small, and the researchers were not truly able to isolate the effects of individual aspects of the intervention.

Mahendra and Arkin (2003) describe a similarly innovative programme where they used students, assistants and volunteers to provide an elder rehabilitation programme. The authors had previously run a programme where volunteers spent two hours per week with patients doing meaningful community activities and verbal fluency or conversation stimulation tasks. The authors found significant improvements in verbal skills, particularly on topic statements and comprehension tasks. The new programme incorporated a physical exercise session into the existing one, using a stationary bike or treadmill, during which memory and conversation stimulation exercises was simultaneously completed with students. The students were provided with ideas and lists of appropriate tasks such as picture or object description, category fluency, pro's and con's discussions, car bingo, etc. Results demonstrated improvements in discourse ratings, proverb comprehension and maintenance of picture description skills over a 4-year period. This is in significant contrast to untreated dementia patients who have been documented in the literature to decline significantly on picture description tasks. However, there were limitations to this study, including the lack of division between tasks, which means there is no clear evidence that it was the combination of tasks that helped rather than just one element. No control group was used and the number of participants was relatively small. Finally, the researchers did not differentiate between dementia groups when they chose their participants, so it is difficult to say how different patients might benefit.

However, these two interventions do demonstrate how volunteers, students and other staff such as assistants can be used in an innovative way to support patients with dementia. The treatment protocols incorporate aspects of both physical and cognitive stimulation, something that perhaps mirrors the work of the multidisciplinary team.

In summary

The individual and group therapies described in this chapter for patients with dementia are not strictly 'impairment'-based therapies at all. However, it is important that the clinician is aware that most of these approaches necessitate knowledge of some aspect of impairment. Simply having an understanding of the individual's areas of cognitive and communication strengths and difficulties will enable you to choose more appropriate communication strategies or aids. For example, recommending the use of appropriate sentence or word complexity to suit the individual's skills for developing a memory or communication aid, and choosing relevant cognitive stimulation tasks, such as verbal fluency or object description tasks in a therapy session.

In short, however, when examining the evidence it becomes obvious that the most robust research into these types of cognitive-communication therapies is in the area of cognitive stimulation therapy groups. Cognitive stimulation therapy groups have been systematically reviewed and researched and are recommended by the NICE guidelines as well as many other organizations. Speech and language therapy input to these types of sessions is essential, although what format this may take can be flexible to suit the needs of both client and clinician. As with many of the approaches outlined in this chapter, setting up a programme that can then be run by others, with supervisory support from yourself would likely be the best use of precious clinical time.

References

Aguirre, E., Spector, A., Streater, A., Hoe, J., Woods, B., and Orrell, M. (2011) *Making a Difference 2*. London: Hawker Publications.

Alm, N., Astell, A., Ellis, M., Dye, R., & Gowans, G. (2004) A cognitive prosthesis and communication support for people with dementia. *Neuropsychological Rehabilitation* 14(1–2) 114–134.

American Speech-Language-Hearing Association (2005) The roles of speech-language pathologists working with individuals with dementia-based communication disorders: Technical report. Available from www.asha.org/policy

Anderson, M., Anzalone, J., Holland, L., & Tracey, E. (2011) Treatment of language, motor speech impairment and dysphagia. *Continuum Lifelong Learning Neurology* 17(3), 471–493.

Arkin, S. & Mahendra, N. (2001) Discourse analysis of Alzheimer's patients before and after intervention methodology and outcomes. *Aphasiology* 15, 533–569.

Baker, J. (2001) How I manage dementia: Living in the real world. *Speech and Language Therapy Practice*. Downloaded from: http://www.speechmag.com/content/files/Microsoft_Word__maryheritage2001.pdf

Black, C. (2005) Speech and language therapy work in Sonas groups. In Marshall, M. *Perspectives of Rehabilitation and Dementia*. London: Jessica Kingsley Publishers.

Bourgeois, M.S. (2007) Memory books and other graphic cuing systmes. New York: Health Professions Press, Brookes.

Bourgeois, M.S. & Hickey, E.M. (2009) *Dementia: From Diagnosis to Management – A Functional Approach*. New York: Psychology Press.

Brown, L. (1997) Activating potential for communication. *Speech & Language Therapy in Practice*. Downloaded from: http://www.speechmag.com/content/files/Sonasapc.pdf

Bruce, E., Hodgson, S., Schweitzer, A., & Schweitzer, P. (1999) *Reminiscing with People with Dementia: A Handbook for Carers*. London: Age Exchange Theatre Trust.

Burgio L.D. & Fisher, S.E. (2000) Application of psychosocial interventions for treating behavioural and psychological symptoms of dementia. *International Psychogeriatrics* 12(1), 351–358.

Cahill, L., Bussolaro, C., Volkmer, A., & Hopkins, K. (2010) Maximizing your memory: Developing a cognitive skills self-management group. Poster Presentation, Melbourne Health Research Week 2010.

Clare, L. & Woods, R.T. (2004) Cognitive training and cognitive rehabilitation for people with early-stage Alzheimer's disease: A review. *Neuropsychological Rehabilitation: An International Journal* 14(4), 385–401.

Connors, T.F. (2000) *Activating the Potential for Communication in People with Dementia in Residential Care. Sonas Model Unit. Project 1*. Dublin: Sonas aPc.

Connors, T.F. (2001) Activating the potential for communication in people with dementia in residential care. Sonas Model Unit. Project 2. Dublin Sonas apc.

Constantinidou, F., Wertheimer, J.C., Tsanadis, J., Evans, C., & Paul, D.R. (2012) Assessment of executive functioning in brain injury: Collaboration between speech-language pathology and neuropsychology for an integrative neuropsychogical perspective. *Brain Injury* 1–15. Posted online 9 July 2012. doi:10.3109/02699052.2012.698786

Cornis-Pop, M., Mashima, P.A., Roth, C.R., Maclennan, D.L., Picon, L.M., Hammond, C.S., Goo-Yashimo, S., Isaki, E., Singson, M., & Frank, E.M. (2012) Cognitive-communication rehabilitation for combat-related mild TBI. *Journal of Rehabilitation Research and Development* **49**(7), xi–xxxi.

Croot, K., Nickels, L., Laurence, F., & Manning, M. (2009) Impairment- and activity/participation-directed interventions in progressive language impairment: Clinical and theoretical issues. *Aphasiology* **23**(2), 125–160.

Ellis, M.P. & Estell, A.J. (2008) A new approach to communicating with people with advanced dementia: A case study of adaptive interaction. In Zeedyk, S. *Promoting Social Interaction for Individuals with Communicative Impairments Making Contact*. London & Philadelphia; Jessica Kingsley Publishers.

Hamill, R. & Connors, T. (2004) Sonas aPc: Activating the potential for communication through multisensory stimulation. In Jones, G. and Miesen, B. (Eds) *Caregiving in Dementia: Research and Applications*. London: Routledge.

Harris, C.L. (Unpublished) The relevance of life history information and the ongoing use of Intensive Interaction with people who have severe dementia. Unpublished MSc Dissertation, University of Bradford.

Joosten-Weyn Bannigh, L., Kessels, R., Rikkert, M., Geleijins-Lanting, C., & Kraaimaat, F. (2008) A cognitive behavioural group therapy for patients diagnosed with mild cognitive impairment and their significant others: Feasibility and preliminary results. *Clinical Rehabilitation* **22**(8), 731–740.

Kagan, A., Black, S.E., Duchan, J.F., Simmons-Mackie, N., & Square, P. (2001) Training volunteers as conversation partners using "supported conversation for adults with aphasia" (SCA): Controlled trial. *Journal of Speech-Language-Hearing Research* **44**(3), 624–638.

Kasl-Godley, J. & Gatz, M. (2000) Psychosocial interventions for individuals with dementia: An integration of theory, therapy, and a clinical understanding of dementia. *Clinical Psychology Review* **20**(6), 755–782.

Kim, E., Cleary, S., Hopper, T., Bayles, K., Mahendra, N., Azuma, T., & Rackley, A. (2006) Evidence-based practice recommendations for working with individuals with dementia: Group reminiscence therapy. *Journal of Medical Speech-Language Pathology* **14**(3), xxiii–xxxiv.

Lock, S., Wilkinson, R., & Bryan, K. (2008) *Supporting Partners of People with Aphasia in Relationships and Conversation*. Milton Keynes: Speechmark.

Lomas, J., Pickard, L., Bester, S., Elbard, H., Finlayson, A., & Zoghaid, C. (1989) The

Communication Effectiveness Index. Development and psychometric evaluation of a functional communication measure for adult aphasia. *Journal of Speech and Hearing Disorders* **54**, 113–124.

Mahendra, N. & Arkin, S. (2003) Effects of four years of exercise, language and social interventions on Alzheimer's Discourse. *Journal of Communication Disorders* **36**, 395–422.

Metternich, B., Schmidke, K., Dykierek, P., & Hull, M (2008) A pilot group therapy for functional memory disorder. *Psychother. Psychosom.* **77**(4), 259–260.

Mueller, A.A. (1993) Maintaining resources by activating the advisory function the elderly: A new concept in the gerontopsychiatry. *Zeitschrift fur Gerontopsychologie and Psychiatrie*, **6**, 119–125.

Murray, L.L. (1998) Longitudinal treatment of primary progressive aphasia: A case study. *Aphasiology* **12**(7), 651–672.

National Collaborating Centre for Mental Health commissioned by the Social Care Institute for Excellence National Institute for Health and Clinical Excellence (revised 2011) The NICE -SCIE Guideline on Supporting People with Dementia and their Carers in Health and Social Care. National Clinical Practice Guideline Number 42 published by The British Psychological Society and Gaskell. Downloaded from: http://www.nice.org.uk/nicemedia/live/10998/30320/30320.pdf

Papp, K.V., Walsh, S.J., & Snyder, P.J. (2009) Immediate and delayed effects of cognitive interventions in healthy elderly: A review of current literature and future directions. *Alzheimer's Dementia* **5**(1), 50–60.

Perrin, T. (1997) The Positive Response Schedule for Severe Dementia. *Aging and Mental Health* **1**(2), 184–191.

Prince, M., Bryce, R., & Ferri, C. (2011) Alzheimer's Disease International, World Alzheimer report the benefits of early diagnosis and intervention. www.alz.co.uk/worldreport2011

Royal College of Speech and Language Therapists (2005) Speech and language therapy provision for people with dementia. RCSLT Position Paper. London: RCSLT: London.. Downloaded from: www.rcslt.org/resources/publications

Segolene, A., Kole, A., & Groft, A. (2008) Empowerment of patients: Lessons from the rare diseases community. *The Lancet* **371**(9629), 2048–2051.

Spector, A. & Orrell, M. (2010) Using a psychosocial model of dementia as a tool to guide clinical practice. *Int Psychogeriatric* **22**(6), 957–965.

Spector, A., Thorgrimsen, L., Woods, B., Royan, L., Davies, S., & Butterworth, M. (2003) Efficacy of an evidence-based cognitive stimulation therapy programme for people with dementia. Randomised controlled trial. *British Journal of Psychiatry* **183**, 248–254.

Threadgold, M. (1995) *Sonas aPc Manual.* Dublin: Sonas aPc.

Threadgold, M. (2002) Sonas aPc: A new lease of life for some. *Sonas apc* **7**, 35–37.

Threadgold, M. & Grennan, S. (2003) Activating potential for communication through all the senses. *Dementia* **2**(2), 277.

Troyer, A., Murphy, K, Anderson, N. Moscovitch, M., & Craik, F. (2008). Changing everyday behaviour in amnestic mild cognitive impairment: A randomised controlled trial. *Neurological Rehabilitation* **18**(1).

Wong, S.B., Anand, R., Chapman, S.B., Rackley, A., & Zientz, J. (2009) When nouns and verbs degrade: Facilitating communication in semantic dementia. *Aphasiology* **23**(2), 286–301.

Woods, B., Aguirre, E., Spector, A.E., & Orrell, M. (2012) Cognitive stimulation to improve cognitive functioning in people with dementia. *Cochrane Database of Systematic Reviews*. *1.2*. The Cochrane Collaboration. Chichester: John Wiley & Sons, Ltd.

6 Therapy and management: Conversation partners

The Cambridge Online Dictionary defines discourse as "communication in speech or writing". But successful communication requires a communication partner to receive the message. Otherwise communication breaks down. And this is just the tip of the iceberg. For unless the two people involved in the exchange are able to communicate a message to one another and receive information in some kind of common method of communication or language there can be no successful exchange.

In this chapter, we examine what speech and language therapists can do to support families and carers in having conversations with people with dementia. There is a relative plethora of evidence in this area of speech and language therapy for people with dementia compared to other approaches. These studies should guide our practice when planning training or education for carers or care staff.

Indeed, it is clear that supporting and educating people in communicating with individuals who have dementia is an important domain of the speech and language therapist's role:

> "The role of the speech and language pathologist is to provide education, support and training to caregivers of persons with dementia from diagnosis right through the end of life state." (Bourgeois & Hickey, 2009)

Why should training be given to caregivers?

When you are planning therapy for a patient with dementia, you need to assess their potential to make gains in treatment. Interventions that aim to improve linguistic accuracy (Chapter 4) may be considered to have limited value in everyday life, since people with progressive language impairments, such as semantic dementia, will experience an inevitable decline in language skills anyway (Wong, Anand, Chapman et al., 2009). For many individuals, their cognitive impairment is also going to limit any carryover (of gains made) to life outside of your therapy sessions. There will (most likely) be none of these limitations in working with caregivers.

People with communication difficulties may be perceived negatively by carers and staff unable to understand the cause of the person's communication difficulty (Murphy, Gray & Cox, 2007). This can cause deterioration in the individual's mood as well as the mood of their carers. Indeed, carers, nurses (Bourgeois & Hickey, 2009) and family members (Clark & Witte, 1995, cited in Bourgeois, Dijkstra, Burgio & Allen, 2004) report that communication difficulties in people with dementia are a source of significant stress. Bourgeois and Hickey (2009) highlight that misconceptions about communication in dementia, as well as unrealistic expectations and frequent conversation breakdown, can lead to these negative feelings, including frustration and difficulties coping with the caregiver burden.

Wong et al. (2009) advocate that targeting conversational effectiveness offers a promising and 'ecologically valuable' intervention method. Conversation partners are more likely to be able to recall, remember and therefore hopefully apply any strategies you may suggest. In other words, training a caregiver in the use of strategies to cue a person who is experiencing word-finding difficulties may be more effective in reducing frustration than commencing a drilling-style naming programme (Tonkovich, 1999). This method may also allow individuals with dementia to connect meaningfully with people in their immediate surroundings well into the late stages of their disease (Wong et al., 2008). Caregivers who are provided with this type of support report improved self-esteem and sense of mastery, resulting in reduced stress and caregiver burden (Bourgeois & Hickey, 2009).

In short, patients with dementia may benefit more in daily life from this more functional type of intervention than from other impairment-based approaches. The people around the person with dementia will also likely benefit from conversation training and education, reducing their stress levels and increasing their understanding of the patient's areas of difficulties. Both these factors can result in reduced care requirements, enabling people to live at home for longer or requiring less support once they are living in residential accommodation.

The following sections discuss training family members and staff in communicating with people with dementia. They outline different approaches including more individualized interventions as well as group-based education and training programmes.

Training family members

Family members are perhaps the most important people in a patient's life; at the start of the disease they are the ones who are adjusting to the change and the shock as much as the patient. But they are also often the most consistent source of support and, consequently, will be ongoing communication partners throughout the person's life. They are the ones who may accompany the person to appointments. Later, they may become the person's carer and at some point be central to decisions about whether an individual will move to a residential facility. Once there, family will likely continue to visit the person, often on a very regular basis.

Communication difficulties can have a significant impact on family members throughout a person's disease. Orange (1991, cited by Perkins, Whitworth & Lesser, 1998) found that in a survey of family members of dementia patients, around half of the respondents noticed a change in their relationship with their loved ones as a direct result of communication difficulties, and reported frustration, loneliness, guilt, embarrassment and social isolation as a consequence. This emphasizes the importance of communication support, advice and education. It cannot be introduced too early or too late, nor be repeated too often. But take note; you may frequently need to refer a family member on for more psychological support if you are unable to meet their needs.

The NICE SCEI guidelines for dementia (2011) state that caregivers should have access to training courses about dementia and communication in the care of people with dementia. Rogers, Holm, Burgio, et al. (2000) recommend that speech and language therapists dedicate at least 5–10 minutes per client per week in the clinic to observing and facilitating communication between clients and their communication partners. However, before rushing to change all your therapy intervention it is worth remembering that all family members are different and have different support needs. Communication support can come in many different shapes and sizes, ranging from telephone support, written materials and books to individual or group training (Bourgeois & Hickey, 2009). Table 6.1 provides a summary of therapy and management ideas for training family members in conversation strategies.

Table 6.1 Therapy/management ideas for training family members in conversation strategies.

Level of impairment	Suggested therapy intervention
Co-morbid difficulties impacting on communication such as hearing and visual impairment either caused by, or alongside, the dementia	Brief education of carers, e.g. basic active listening strategies Onward referral for audiology, ophthalmology, optometry assessment or other allied health input
Progressive language impairment (e.g. svPPA) or primarily communication difficulties with little cognitive impairment	Written information leaflets from the Alzheimer's society website Individualized education and conversation training within therapy sessions using models such as SPPARC Group-based support or education sessions
Complex cognitive communication difficulties resulting from a mixture of reduced memory, poor self-monitoring, reduced insight, impaired executive skills, etc	Written information leaflets from the Alzheimer's society website Individualized education and conversation training Group-based support or education sessions
Profound global communication and cognitive impairment	Group-based support or education sessions Individual training to use strategies such as the Sonas aPc or intensive interaction type approaches (Chapter 5)

Is individual or group education more useful?

Perkins et al. (1998) describe conversation as a joint responsibility and dependent not just on the patient's strengths or weaknesses but the interactional strengths and weaknesses of two people. Consequently, prior to setting up any training or education sessions it is important to understand the dynamics of a conversation between the patient and their loved one. In comparison with conversation between the therapist and the person with dementia, conversation with a loved one may be quite different. This doesn't mean that conversation will necessarily be more difficult with family members. Perkins et al. (1998) cite Ramanthan-Abbott (1994) who found that patients with dementia often communicate with less difficulty with spouses than with an unfamiliar conversation partner. This emphasizes the value of having a good understanding of the conversational dynamic between a patient and their loved ones.

Discourse analysis and conversation analysis have been discussed previously (Chapter 2). The following elaborates on this introduction to conversation analysis, particularly focusing on the areas of turn taking, repair and topic maintenance. However, understanding factors that impact on a conversation may involve not only observation of a conversation between the patient and their loved one, but also getting to know the family member's perspective. Engaging a family member in a discussion about the patient's communication strengths and areas of difficulty (using either formal or informal approaches such as the La Trobe communication questionnaire (Douglas et al., 2000)) can provide information on how the family member perceives that person, their understanding of dementia and its impact on communication as well as how they are coping with it themselves.

Having an understanding of both the patient and their family member's areas of concerns can provide information on whether individual or group sessions might be more useful for them. Individual therapy sessions can be more detailed and specific, and be more effective in engaging both the patient and their family member. In comparison, a group can ensure you meet the needs of more people, and can also provide emotional support and problem-solving strategies from other relatives or carers living with similar difficulties (Taylor, Kingma, Croot & Nickels, 2009). The group dynamics can, at times, provide a more powerful support tool compared to the relationship with the therapist. It is important to remember, however, that there will be people who do not like to participate in groups

There are a number of groups that have been described in the literature for relatives of people with dementia. These groups tend to focus on advising families of a variety of communication strategies that might be useful for them when communicating with their loved ones. The most common strategies that clinicians suggest are using short simple sentences and speaking slowly (Small & Gutman, 2002). Other authors, however, have reported carer dissatisfaction with these types of strategies (Orange, 1995, cited by Perkins et al., 1998). There is, in fact, little research into the effectiveness of these types of strategies in real-life situations.

It is also important to acknowledge that running groups effectively is a skill so I would highly recommend attending a group facilitation training session of some sort. More often, the main barrier to setting up a group is not having enough carers or relatives on a caseload who are able to attend at any one time. Perhaps these issues can be easily dealt with, but if not, are you able to set up an evening group, or can you invite relatives or carers of people who have already been discharged? Can you mix relatives of progressive and non-progressive patients? Relatives may or may not cope well with this type of group combination. You must very carefully consider how you will structure any group session, as well as which carers or family members you will invite.

Individual conversation analysis and training sessions

As mentioned above, a period of therapy focusing on conversation training can commence with an assessment of conversation. It is useful for this to be discussed at length here (as well as in Chapter 2), as information from this evaluation will be directly linked to the identification and development of communication strategies. Furthermore, conversation analysis allows both the patient and/or conversation partner to understand and identify areas of difficulty, thereby increasing awareness and insight into the causes of conversation breakdown. Conversation analysis can also act as a method of practising and demonstrating the effectiveness of newly-identified strategies (Perkins et al., 1998).

Conversation analysis and therapy approaches may be familiar to clinicians used to working with non-progressive aphasics. In fact, there are some well-known resources such as Supported Conversation for Adults with Aphasia (Kagan, Black, Duchan, et al., 2001) and the Supporting Partners of People with Aphasia in Relationships and Conversation (SPPARC) approach (Lock, Wilkinson & Bryan, 2001). Although there is no formal research in the use of these approaches with people with progressive language difficulties, they can be modified to suit the needs of these clients. These resources provide a well-structured, systematic method for applying conversation analysis as a therapeutic process that focuses on areas of conversation such as breakdown and repair, turn taking and topic maintenance. These approaches require the dyad to make a video recording of a typical conversation. The patient and their partner are then encouraged to participate in the evaluation of this video. Other authors have also focused on these three areas – topic maintenance, repair and turn taking – in relation to communication breakdown for people with dementia (such as Perkins et al., 1998). Table 6.2 provides a summary of some potential areas of difficulty for people with dementia across these domains. This description also briefly highlights which strategies may or may not be useful in these instances.

Table 6.2 Potential areas of difficulty and strategies for people with dementia across the areas of turn taking, repair and topic maintenance.

Domain	Potential areas of difficulty and strategies
Turn taking	This is a mechanical aspect of communication, which is preserved in dementia but can be cognitively difficult due to, for example, delayed processing which means it is more difficult to hold on to a turn. This can result in patients taking more passive roles and initiating conversation less. Other deficits such as reduced attention can make it hard to respond appropriately to questions or comments. Word-finding difficulties and reduced comprehension can also contribute to this difficulty. People with communication difficulties resulting from dementia may leave large gaps mid-turn, which conversation partners can misinterpret. The conversation partner's skills in timing, giving adequate time to answer, or changing topics can also pose a difficulty for the individual with dementia. Hamilton (1994) describes how people with aphasia and people with Alzheimer' disease will often use strategies to maintain a turn, such as minimal turns 'hmmm', 'aha', 'yeah' and 'OK'. These strategies can support the flow of conversation and act in a range of communicative functions.
Repair	Repair allows you to deal with breakdown and for conversation to continue. Perkins et al. (1998) highlight that breakdown may not occur simply when the person with dementia makes an error, as would be expected from the results of a more formal assessment of communication (where any errors would be scored as breakdown). Perkins et al. cite Schlegoff et al. (1977) who analyzed normal conversational repair and broke it up into: – self initiated repair – other initiated repair – self repair – other repair Self-initiated self-repair is considered most 'normal'. Hamilton (1994) found that in early- and mid-stage dementia repair is often self-initiated and sometimes self-repaired. In mid- to late-stage dementia repair is more likely just to be ignored or abandoned, even if the listener attempts to initiate and assist this process. This can result in increased conversation breakdown. It can be assumed, suggest Perkins et al. (1998), that the less impairment the person has the more easily they will be able to self-repair. Yet, equally, someone who is less impaired may choose to avoid trying to repair to 'save face', as this attempt would reveal how difficult this is for him or her. Later on in their illness, however, it becomes more likely that the individual with dementia is simply unaware of the errors they make. It is therefore worth considering the value of repairing conversation breakdown; it could be more awkward in conversation if every breakdown was constantly highlighted to a patient who is already embarrassed by their condition. Appropriate strategies will therefore need to be mutually agreed. And family members may feel less frustrated if they understand the reason why their relative is not trying to make repairs in conversation.

(Continued overleaf)

Topic maintenance	Topic maintenance involves taking turns to talk through a topic. Perkins et al. (1998) highlight that this can become difficult for people with dementia due to language impairments, but also reduced attention, judgement, memory, confabulations and other cognitive difficulties. Topic use may be characterized by reduced topic initiation, but also inappropriately frequent topic shifts without closing previous topics. Hamilton (1994) suggests that it is particularly difficult for people with dementia to perceive other people's points of view and therefore this impacts on their ability to judge topic change. This means it can become the unimpaired conversation partner's responsibility to repair and maintain conversational topic relevance.

The SPPARC model describes how patients and communication partners can participate in creating and evaluating a video of themselves in conversation, identifying areas of strength and difficulty (such as strategies that worked well, or failed) and then problem solving how to improve this interaction, before trialing strategies together. This is described as a group intervention for people with non-progressive aphasia. This approach has also been used to effect in individual therapy with non-progressive aphasics (Volkmer, 2006). Such an approach could be applied to a progressive population. Indeed, researchers and clinicians often report introducing using video feedback to support the introduction of communications aids and total communication strategies with relatives of patients with dementia (Murray, 1998).

Another model of providing assessment and feedback through conversation analysis is the Conversation Analysis Profile for People with Cognitive Impairment (CAPPCI) developed by Perkins, Whitworth and Lesser (1997). This model of assessment and intervention requires first of all an interview with the caregiver as well as an analysis of a sample of conversation. This information is analyzed and combined to provide a profile of what is occurring in interaction. This then supports the planning of appropriate therapy tasks to improve interaction. The interview with the caregiver focuses on asking them to rate the frequency of different behaviours. It also allows the clinician to gather information about the types of strategies the caregiver feels they are using, as well as how successful these are in practice. The interview attempts to identify whether the carer feels each of the identified behaviours is causing a problem. Finally, the interview also asks about pre-dementia versus current communication styles and opportunities for communication. This can guide the amount of education the carer may benefit from. It will also illustrate how carers have accepted behaviours and whether they may be underestimating their partner's skills. Therapists can reinforce successful strategy use or discourage unsuccessful strategies by comparing what carers say works to the conversation sample, as well as highlighting unnoticed strategies and suggest new ones too.

What does the evidence tell us?

A brief review of the literature tells us that there has been relatively little work done around conversation analysis with people with dementia, and what has been done focuses mainly on using rating scales rather than conversational samples. For a fuller description of methods of conversational analysis with people with dementia it is worth referring back to Chapter 2.

In terms of therapy approaches for conversation training, there is little evidence in the literature on patients with dementia. The most useful and applicable examples come from some case studies such as 'DD' described by Murray (1998) and 'Bobby V' described by Wong et al. (2009). Both of these have been described in Chapter 5 when discussing interventions to increase patient self-monitoring and awareness. In this chapter, we describe how the authors focused on training the patient's spouses.

Murray (1998) describes how she highlighted to DD and her spouse the turn taking and repair strategies they were already using (based on pre-treatment conversational samples). They discussed the effectiveness of these strategies as well as possible alternatives. Murray then staged role-play sessions with DD, modelling target alternatives which were videotaped. These videotapes were later examined and discussed by DD, her spouse and the author. Following this, further role-play, PACE tasks and videotape review were used to model and elicit specific strategies designed to facilitate interactions. One example of this was demonstrating to DD's spouse the effectiveness of requests for elaboration from DD when he did not understand her, rather than asking her to repeat what she had said. After this period of therapy, re-evaluation of the couple's conversation demonstrated increased repertoire and use of repair strategies. And DD demonstrated improvements and maintained performance on communication measures including the CADL and the CETI and high ratings on the ASHA FACS.

Wong et al. (2009) used information from analyzing the discourse between their case study, 'Bobby V' and his wife, to provide training to his wife. They started by explaining the effect of his communication difficulties on his conversation and how this may present as his apparent 'egotism'. They encouraged her to focus on the message as a whole rather than insisting on lexical specificity. They highlighted the association between a number of his stereotyped phrases and the particular contexts, such as the fact that he used the phrase 'that's kind of flaky' to compensate for his poor verbal description or his behaviour. They suggested she could use this knowledge to prompt herself to clarify his underlying meaning at these times. They also highlighted her role as a liaison between Bobby V and other conversation partners, to act as a conversational ramp; providing words, clarifying his message and accepting his conversational turns in wider social situations. One method of supporting the use of these strategies was to trial their use in the conversation group they were attending. Wong et al. (2009) suggest that their discourse intervention probably facilitated Bobby V's success in participating in conversation rather than withdrawing due to frustration. Helping his wife focus on residual abilities also enabled them to maintain meaningful interactions. The authors reported a change in her perception; where previously she had considered him egotistical, she now felt less frustrated by his communication difficulties. However, the authors emphasize the limitations to this approach, one of which is the lack of evidence about how long these positive effects will be maintained.

Group education and conversation training

There are a number of examples of group education and conversation training groups that have been developed for relatives and carers of people with dementia. These often take the form of quite traditional teaching and workshop sessions such as the FOCUSED programme. FOCUSED is a communication skills training programme designed by Ripich, Ziol, Fritsch and Durand (1994) for nursing staff. However, it has also been modified to suit the needs of families. The sessions typically run for one or two hours per week over four to eight weeks. FOCUSED training is presented by a speech and language therapist using the FOCUSED programme but includes discussion questions, videotaped vignettes, role-play activities, a caregiver's guide and prompt card. This is a seven-step programme teaching specific conversation skills under the following headings:

> Face: face the person, call his name, touch him, gain and maintain eye contact.
>
> Orient: orient the person to the topic by repeating key words several times, repeat and rephrase sentences, use nouns and specific names.
>
> Continue: continue the same topic of conversation for as long as possible, restate the topic throughout the conversation, indicate to the person that you are introducing a new topic .

Un-stick: help the person become 'unstuck' when he or she uses a word incorrectly by suggesting the intended word, repeat the sentence the person said using the correct word, ask 'Do you mean '...' ?'

Structured: structure your questions so the person will be able to recognize and repeat a response, provide two simple choices at a time, use yes/no questions.

Exchange: keep up the normal exchange of ideas used in everyday conversation, keep conversations going with comments such as 'Oh how nice', or 'That's great', do not ask test questions, give the person clues as to how to answer your questions.

Direct: keep sentences short, simple and direct, put the subject of the sentences first, use and repeat nouns (names) rather than pronouns (he, she, it), use hand signals, pictures and facial expressions.

(See Table 6.3 for a list of suggested strategies to support conversation training.)

Patient-centered self-management groups have also become increasingly popular in many chronic conditions including dementia. We described in detail an example of a patient education group in the previous chapter (Cahill, Bussolaro, Volkmer & Hopkins, 2010). This group involved both patients and their carers or relatives in the same group and required both parties to set goals prior to attending. This meant that the groups could be tailored to all participants needs. There was a focus on a number of different topics but the study included developing communication skills over a series of sessions. Including both people with dementia and their relatives meant that both parties were aware of strategies and information being given and reported having a better understanding of the other person's perspective. Results demonstrated that almost all goals were achieved. Where the goals were not addressed (e.g. continence management), this person could be referred on for further individualized sessions to address ongoing concerns (Cahill et al., 2010).

There are many other examples of group programmes outside of the National Health Service for relatives of people with dementia. These are often designed for certain disease groups and may be provided by organizations such as charities and universities. One example is described by the Northwestern University in Chicago, who set up a group programme for patients and relatives of people with PPA. They aimed to provide specific feedback and education to improve communication between patients with PPA and their families (Cognitive Neurology and Alzheimer's Disease Centre (CNADC), Northwestern University Chicago, 2002). There are also groups such as the Frontotemporal Dementia Support Group in the UK, which runs on a quarterly basis to provide support and invites professionals to the sessions (http://www.ftdsg.org/ Frontotemporal dementia support group). Being aware of the services provided by local branches of the Alzheimer's Society, frontotemporal dementia support groups, Admiral Nursing (in some parts of the UK) or other local charities can provide can be useful for you and your patients.

Table 6.3 Suggested strategies to support conversation training (some of which have come from Smith & Buckwater, 2005; NICE guidelines, 2011; Fels & Astell, 2011; as well as from clinical experience).

Strategies to support conversation training
Talking to people with dementia • Before you start communication, get the person's attention, make eye contact, and speak directly to the person (unless this is culturally inappropriate). • Ensure that people with sensory impairments have eyeglasses, hearing aids, and adequate lighting; without them, misinterpretations of stimuli can lead to behavioural or psychological symptoms. • Provide guidance to minimize surprises. For example, when approaching a person with dementia, a staff member should first identify her or himself and address the patient by name, then explain in simple terms what she will be doing. A silent approach from behind can be unnecessarily frightening. • Non-verbal communication is very useful for people with dementia, particularly tone of voice, facial expressions, and use of non-verbal gestures (for example, showing the person how to brush her teeth while saying "Brush your teeth"). • Slow down the pace of speech, using short sentences, and using nouns (chair, bathroom) instead of pronouns (it, there). • Avoid commands that include the word 'don't' and questions that begin with 'why'. Which may prevent the patient feeling that they are being reprimanded or tested. • Breaking down tasks into steps, while providing encouragement and reassurance, helps the person to act as independently as possible. Well-meaning but misguided caregivers can worsen anxiety and frustration by asking the person to 'try harder' (for example, "You did it yesterday; what's the problem today?" or "If you wanted to, you could do it."). • Use language that is non-discriminatory and positive, i.e. do not compare the person's performance to others on the unit, do not make comments related to their age, focus on how well they are managing.

- It's common to rephrase a question a person doesn't understand but this could actually increase confusion. Instead, ask only one question at a time, allow time for a response, and repeat the question if needed.

- Confronting delusions or confabulations with facts is not reassuring. For example, instead of responding to someone who says she is expecting her father to visit with "Your father is dead", it may be better to distract her by reminiscing with her about her childhood. Some staff may feel uncomfortable with this approach, feeling that they are lying if they do not answer questions like this directly. However, it may be more appropriate to use a re-orientation approach when you have more time to provide appropriate reassurance, as guided by the psychologist working with the particular client.

- Monitor and adjust the environment. Simple adjustments, such as placing a clock and calendar in the room, may help those still oriented to time and place. Family photographs on walls and shelves, familiar furniture and ornaments can allow them to reminisce in day-to-day conversation with carers and staff. Large signs, pictures, or coloured arrows can help people find their way around their own home or a facility, or even remind them of where particular kitchen items are stored.

Understanding people with dementia

- People with dementia may say or do things that caregivers and staff don't understand or that they find silly and annoying. It's easy to view these behaviours as meaningless, yet they may be better understood as attempts to communicate. For example, a tendency to repeat questions is common in people with dementia, so in this instance it is important to try to detect the real message. Someone who repeatedly asks, "When is lunch?" may be hungry or thirsty and should be offered food or drink.

- Similarly, a patient may try to engage in behaviours such as leaving the building, stating they have to "go to work" after 20 years of retirement or wish to look for someone who has been dead for decades. Engaging in an activity such as gardening, food preparation, or reminiscence may provide a distraction. Engaging in these type of activities early, rather than ignoring behaviours or hoping they will stop on their own, can avoid more intense and discomforting behaviours.

- Patients with dementia can engage in the same story-telling process as they did before they had dementia. However, a critical part of this story telling is the listener. Supportive or attentive listeners who collaborate with the story teller using specific phrases such as 'uhhuh', 'really', 'that's interesting' encourage participants to continue. This means not doing other things at the same time and not giving their own anecdotes. Story telling with stories from the past that do not have to be 'correct' allow patients to produce 'tell-able' tales.

What does the evidence tell us?

In general, there are very few reviews of training programmes that specifically examine support given to improve communication skills for family members, probably because the literature focuses more on counselling, coping and social support (Ripich et al., 1998). What evidence there is, however, is much easier to find than other literature on therapy approaches for people with dementia. This is perhaps due to the crossover between conversation training for family members and nursing staff. Many of the programmes for caregivers or families have been adapted from programmes designed for nursing staff. Ripich, for example, designed the FOCUSED programme for nursing staff before it was trialled with family members and caregivers.

Ripich et al. (1998) described training 19 caregivers (family members and spouses) of people with mid-stage Alzheimer's disease using the FOCUSED programme and compared this group to a control group of family members and carers who received no input. Results showed that FOCUSED group participants rated communication 'hassles' as having decreased over time, whilst knowledge about Alzheimer's disease increased. This was reviewed at 12 months following the training, and improvements were maintained. In short, understanding communication breakdown in Alzheimer's' disease and learning how to cope with these results reduced the care burden for relatives of people with dementia. The authors hypothesize that caregivers require time to practise and integrate information and strategies before they can have an impact on conversation. They suggest that this development in the successful implementation of strategies also supports the ongoing use of strategies and therefore maintenance of results at 12 months. It is valuable to note, however, that many of the strategies used in this programme are those that have been found not to be useful in other research which surveyed the perceived usefulness of a series of strategies by caregivers and family members (Small & Gutman, 2002). This probably highlights the importance of individualized approaches even when planning a group intervention.

Ripich, Ziol, Fritsch and Durand (1999) continued their research into the use of the FOCUSED programme with 32 caregivers of people with dementia. The caregivers attended training over four weekly one-hour sessions They were able to demonstrate specific improvements in the types of questions used by carers, particularly the use of more closed questions and the consequent increase in successful responses from the person they cared for. They also introduced booster groups, which resulted in little maintenance of skills when compared with those who did not attend booster groups. They suggest that future maintenance might be best enhanced though more personally relevant support. This echoes some of the previous comments highlighted by Small and Gutman (2002).

Other types of group training and support have also been shown to reduce carer burden in partners of people with dementia. Established in 1995,

Resources for Enhancing Alzheimer's Caregiver Health (REACH) is a unique, multisite research programme. The researchers developed and evaluated a variety of multicomponent interventions for family caregivers of persons with Alzheimer's disease at the mild or moderate level of impairment. Six different interventions were trialled across six different sites in America. These included: (a) Individual Information and Support Strategies; (b) Group Support and Family Systems Therapy; (c) Psycho-educational and Skill-Based Training Approaches; (d) Home-Based Environmental Interventions; and (e) Enhanced Technology Support Systems. Each intervention required specific training and a handbook was provided to ensure consistency in provision. At a 6-month evaluation, active interventions, whatever the type, were considered superior to control conditions in relation to carer burden (Gitlin, Burgio, Czaja, Mahoney, et al., 2003). This suggests that some patients may benefit equally from group communication training as from other types of group interventions.

The NICE guidelines for dementia (2011) include a brief review of a number of group education and support groups focusing predominantly on psychological support groups for carers. This report suggests that, in general, interventions involving training and stress management or involving the person with dementia alongside the carer appeared to have the largest effect on the carer's psychological health and wellbeing. Carers also benefit from support groups where they can learn from one another and the group, groups which can provide education and information with support from local services. In short, it may be useful to collaborate with other disciplines or other providers (such as support groups) before setting up your own group programme. Perhaps providing a communication skills training session as part of a larger programme could be more useful.

See Case Study 3 in Chapter 5 (Mr F) for an example of how a carer education group can support a patient and his relatives.

Training nursing staff and other professionals

Communication breakdown is consistently highlighted as one of the most stressful problems faced by carers of people with Alzheimer's disease (Ripich et al., 1998). This highlights the stress and difficulties that staff may experience day in and day out when working with people with dementia in nursing and residential homes, on wards and when attending them in their own homes.

There is also a growing awareness that the way that people interact and communicate with patients with dementia can significantly influence how that individual behaves. This means that certain types of communication can trigger 'problem behaviour' whilst other communication styles may also help manage that behaviour (Burgio & Fisher, 2000). Indeed, the quality of staff members' communication with patients with dementia has been shown to have a major impact on patients' quality of life (CSCI, 2008, cited by Department of Health, 2009).

Thankfully, regular communication training is becoming commonplace for nursing and care staff. Indeed, the NICE guidelines 2011 state that:

> "While many care staff have high levels of skill and expertise, they need help and support to develop these skills, with communication with people with dementia being a particular area where there is a need for training."

Providing training is integral to the speech and language therapists' core role, "as outcomes for people with speech, language and communication needs are improved when the whole workforce is able to contribute appropriately to care pathways" (RCSLT, 2009). Table 6.4 gives a list of ideas for training nursing staff, carers and other professionals in conversation strategies.

Table 6.4 Therapy/management ideas for training nursing staff, carers and other professionals in conversation strategies.

Level of difficulty	Suggested therapy intervention
Patient is having difficulties following some basic instructions in therapy or care activities. Staff are asking for advice to guide them in managing specific tasks with patients such as doing physiotherapy, or completing a wash and dressing routine	Communication passports Coaching and observation, co-facilitation of groups and sessions Communication aids and life review books to support conversations
Patient is verbal or non-verbal but may have some significant cognitive, communication and behavioural difficulties that affect all aspects of their day. This may be similar to a number of people in the unit/ward/residential setting. Staff are seeking advice to guide them in everyday interactions, a reminder and update on best practice	More formal training and education sessions, including the use of mentorship and rewarded learning
Patient is almost non-verbal. Staff are unsure if the patient can communicate at all and find they barely interact with the patient	Specific one-to-one training of staff in approaches to maximize communication awareness, e.g. use of Intensive interaction

Understanding how other staff members work

When working with other staff members it is important to remember that nursing and care staff in particular spend most of their time with the patients we are speaking to them about. These staff members are experts in providing care to these individuals on a daily basis and know them well. They are often able to reflect on the most useful approaches to communication through their own experience but at other times they may need some support.

It can be valuable to become more aware of the models of care that nursing staff are using in your facility to guide you when planning a training session. Smith and Buckwater (2005) describe two models of care used in nursing. Both models are based on the belief that psychological and behavioural symptoms in dementia are a form of communication.

The Progressively Lowered Stress Threshold Model was developed in response to observations of patients with Alzheimer disease. According to this model, adults with dementia become less able to manage stress as the disease progresses. That is, their 'stress threshold' becomes lower, resulting in anxiety and increasingly dysfunctional behaviours. Stressors may include what we would consider routine aspects of daily life: fatigue; changes in routine or staff members; environmental triggers; overwhelming information; grief; illness; pain, etc. They suggest six essential principles of care using this model. This includes strategies to modify the environment, provision of 'unconditional positive regard', observation of anxiety and avoidance in patients to guide activities and promoting comfort and function, by understanding and managing personal, social, and physical factors that may trigger behaviours.

The Need-Driven Dementia-Compromised Behavior Model, developed in 1993, suggests that 'disruptive' or 'disturbing' behaviours are potentially understandable needs. If these needs are responded to appropriately, a person's quality of life may be enhanced. In this model, behavioural symptoms are considered to be the result of complex interactions between 'background' and 'proximal' factors. Background factors are more individual and disease-related factors, such as marital status, personality traits, overall health status and language impairment. Proximal factors are those that precipitate a particular disruptive or disturbing behaviour such as an unmet physiological need (e.g. hunger), an unmet psychosocial need (contact with friends), a disturbing environmental issue (a cold room), or uncomfortable social surroundings (too many people in a room). In this model, proximal factors guide the development of nursing interventions.

If you are aware of the model of care, the level of knowledge and areas of need for the team you are working with, you will be better able to plan the most appropriate training package. Do not hesitate to ask the team what they need. Staff can often tell you exactly what would be most useful. And, similarly to our patients, are consequently more likely to engage.

Planning a training session

Supporting our colleagues in communicating with patients can take many different forms because of the needs of the patient or the staff members. This may include acting in a type of 'coaching role'. Coaching typically involves observing colleagues in practice, and consequently providing either verbal suggestions or jointly facilitating a session to model strategies that work with a particular individual or group of patients. This can be especially useful for complex clients or when supporting staff members to facilitate groups (Tonkovich, 1999). Bourgeois and Hickey (2009) have identified this type of training as being of particular value to staff and patients when introducing communication and memory aids or life review books in facilities such as nursing homes.

Traditionally, training of staff members has focused on more didactic teaching sessions, which are now more often facilitated in a workshop style. FOCUSED is a communication skills training programme designed by Ripich et al. (1994) for nursing staff working with people with dementia. It has also been modified to suit the needs of families, and was described in detail earlier in this chapter. The sessions typically run for one or two hours per week over 6–8 weeks. FOCUSED training is presented by a speech and language therapist using the FOCUSED programme but includes discussion questions, videotaped vignettes, role-play activities, a written guide and prompt card. See Table 6.5 for suggestions of how to structure a teaching session for carers or staff members.

In-service teaching and on-the-job training (or coaching) may be accompanied by motivational systems that incorporate rewards and corrective feedback. In some UK health trusts, motivational systems such as these have been linked with mandatory training schemes, contribution towards qualifications such as recognized national vocational qualifications or have been rewarded through ongoing supervision, appraisal and management systems. Other trusts have invited nursing homes to pay towards training schemes, which has resulted in improved participant attendance and improved perception of value of training.

However, supporting our colleagues may not always be so hands-on and could involve the provision of specific information such as a communication passport or specific communication guidelines. This type of written guidance can flag certain strategies that support interactions with specific patients, and can easily be passed on to new staff members. See Table 6.4 for a list of suggested conversation strategies that can be integrated into training sessions or communication passports.

Table 6.5 Structuring a teaching session with carers or staff members.

Introductions/ aims	Introductions can be formal for a larger group or informal for a smaller. For example, pass a ball or bean bag around the group and state a personal piece of information such as favourite colour, or how long it took to travel to meeting. Can make it physical to increase interaction and ask people to stand in order of distance travelled (to do this they have to start talking to one another!).
	Can give aims, or ask attendees what they would like to know/find useful. This can be done in advance or on the day.
Communication difficulties in dementia	It can be helpful to:
	• present information on dementia – a medical definition, for example (invite people, e.g. medical staff psychologist, to present this section with you to give emphasis)
	• present information on how this affects communication, e.g. using a model of language processing if you are focusing on language
	• define different communication difficulties such as dysarthria, dysphasia, dsypraxia and cognitive communication as well as highlight that hearing and vision can impact on communication
	• list cognitive communication and language, and link this to the neuroanatomy of dementia
	• invite attendees to give examples of how conversation breaks down for patients, and share their stories or experiences
	• use current case examples of patients on the ward or unit to help staff, or video clips or vignettes to assist them in identifying or observing communication difficulties
	• break into smaller groups and use written scenarios where group attendees need to identify communication difficulties
	• understand how communication difficulties might feel – putting themselves in the patient with dementia's position, e.g. asking one person in a pair to communicate a message without using any word with an 'e' in it. Or asking one person in the pair how it feels to try to understand what someone is saying who is not allowed to use words at all to give an instruction
	• link theory to policies, e.g. NICE guidelines or trust policies

(Continued overleaf)

Strategies	It can be helpful to: • invite attendees to provide examples and share strategies they use with patients/relatives • invite attendees to think about how conversation in normal life works, e.g. what do they do when they can't hear someone, or the room is busy, or if someone has not understood them • invite attendees to observe vignettes acted by facilitator or on video to aid reflection process and identify what worked or didn't work and what might work better next time. The facilitators may then act the same scenario using the identified strategies successfully, or you can invite participants to act out the scenario using strategies • give attendees a written scenario to work on in pairs to identify strategies that may have worked better • provide a list of strategies to the group (it may often be most helpful to do this at the end of the session using only strategies and wording that the group has generated)
Practice	It can be helpful to provide participants with assignments to complete in the interval or between group sessions, such as writing down some of the communication difficulties they may observe, or using a specific strategy with a patient or their loved ones and feeding back to the group
Finish and follow-up	It is important to finish a group with a specific exercise or task, such as a relaxing cup of tea and cake and an opportunity to chat with one another or the facilitator. It can also be an exercise such as: • a thank you, where each person says thank you for something specific to do with the session, or chooses a picture from a selection that they feel best represents their experience in the group and explaining/sharing it with the group • asking participants to identify one thing that they have learned or one thing they will do to change their practice, and write it down or announce it to the group • holding a follow-up group a few weeks after the final session to find out how people are progressing • meet people individually to either observe how they are coping, or discuss any goals or outcome measures may need to be reviewed Information can also be linked into performance management or appraisal with the managers of staff; there is evidence that staff who are rewarded for maintaining their skills continue to practice them
Evaluation	It is always important to evaluate your group using either written or verbal feedback. This can be immediate or come later (e.g. via post), asking advice on what was or was not useful and what to change for the future.

What does the evidence tell us?

The research into training staff who work with people with dementia is generally focused on nursing staff and nursing assistants and is overwhelmingly positive. The main barriers to this type of training have been about maintaining the gains people have made in daily practice, and studies have started to address these problems through analysis of motivational systems. The NICE guidelines, however, remind clinicians that there are limitations to the research that can be conducted in nursing or residential homes with people with dementia due to the high attrition rate of participants (referring to the high mortality rate in severe dementia), but also the high rates of staff turnover.

The FOCUSED programme has been mentioned previously in this chapter when describing the research that has been done in the area of caregiver training. Ripich et al.'s FOCUSED programme was, however, initially designed with nursing staff in mind. Ripich et al. (1998) describe how 17 nursing assistants were trained using the FOCUSED programme. The study demonstrated that nursing assistants showed increased control over social interaction and improved satisfaction in social interaction with people with Alzheimer's disease. Burgio and Fisher (2000) describe a number of previous studies that examined training of nursing assistants. All of these demonstrated positive outcomes in the reduction of aggressive behaviour on the units, and improved coping and less frustration reported by staff (Hoeffer et al., 1997 and McCallion et al., 1999). The NICE guidelines (2011) also describe the study by McCallion et al. (1999) where nursing aides were taught a communication skills programme which resulted in positive outcomes, including a reduction in the staff turnover rates and improved staff knowledge of care-giving responses.

Burgio and Fisher (2000) went on to complete a number of studies comparing teaching tools used in training staff. This included in-services, on-the-job training, and a motivational system incorporating rewards and corrective feedback. Results demonstrated improved communication; particularly verbal prompting, announcing an activity, use of one-step instructions and pauses, and use of diverting techniques. However, only staff members who were then supported with the staff motivational systems maintained their skills up to 46 months later. The NICE guidelines (2011) also describe a number of studies that examined the effect of staff training on both behaviour management and communication skills with patients with dementia. All these studies indicate that training which is supported by ongoing work place shadowing, joint working and formal staff management support systems is more successful in maintaining skills learned in the initial training sessions.

This summary of work highlights the undoubtedly positive impact that communication training can have for patients, but also emphasizes the need for us as clinicians to consider how we will ensure the maintenance of these skills. The NICE guidelines (2011) highlight that measuring the impact of this type of intervention in practice may need to focus on more qualitative information such as improvements in health professionals' behaviour management rather than the impact on a patient. Although they stress this should have a knock-on effect on enhancing care and wellbeing in patients it is difficult to measure this outcome in the clinical setting. Clinicians do need to reflect the effectiveness and outcomes of staff training packages, so using qualitative measures during sessions such as questionnaires and staff reported outcome measures is supported by this literature.

In summary

The purpose of conversation-focused intervention in dementia is to maintain an optimum level of communication and social connectedness. Yet discourse requires the joint construction of a message by a listener and a speaker. This means that as clinicians we need to involve both the patient and their communication partner (Wong et al., 2009). This should include working with family caregivers or staff members either in people's homes or in residential and nursing home settings. Although many clinicians may find it daunting and frustrating working with these groups, it is a part of our role as experts in communication to equip conversation partners with the skills they need (Bourgeois & Hickey, 2009; RCSLT Position Paper, 2005).

In practice, it is likely that this type of training will focus on individual training for patients' relatives and more group-based training schemes for staff members. However, it is not simply the conversation training that we must consider. We must bear in mind the burden of working and living with people with cognitive communication difficulties. There are many organizations that can provide support within and outside the national health system for families of people with dementia. This burden can also take its toll on staff, and following up training sessions with ongoing support systems to ensure maintenance of skills has been shown to be effective.

References

Bourgeois, M.S. & Hickey, E.M. (2009) *Dementia: from Diagnosis to Management: A Functional Approach*. New York: Psychology Press.

Bourgeois, M.S., Dijkstra, K., Burgio, L.D., & Allen, R.S. (2004) Communication skills training for nursing aides of residents with dementia: The impact of measuring performance. *Clinical Gerentologist* 27(1/2), 119–128.

Burgio L.D. & Fisher, S.E. (2000) Application of psychosocial interventions for treating behavioural and psychological symptoms of dementia. *International Psychogeriatrics* 12(1), 351–358.

Cahill, L., Bussolaro, C., Volkmer, A., & Hopkins, K. (2010) Maximizing your memory: Developing a cognitive skills self-management group. Poster Presentation.

Cambridge online dictionary (downloaded 2012) http://dictionary.cambridge.org/dictionary/british/discourse?q=discourse

Cognitive Neurology and Alzheimer's Disease Centre (CNADC), Northwestern University Chicago (2012) Primary Progressive Aphasia (PPA) Clinical Program. Viewed online January 2013 at: http://brain.northwestern.edu/dementia/ppa/ppa.html

Department of Health (2009) Living well with dementia: A National Dementia Strategy. Downloaded from: www.dh.gov.uk/prod_consum_dh/groups/dh_digitalassets/@dh/@en/documents/digitalasset/dh_094051.pdf

Douglas, J.M., O'Flaherty, C.A., & Snow, P.C. (2000) Measuring perception of communicative ability: The development and evaluation of the La Trobe Communication Questionnaire. *Aphasiology* 14(3), 251–268.

Fels, D.I. & Astell, A.J. (2011) Storytelling as a model of conversation for people with dementia and caregivers. *Alzheimer's Disease and Other Dementias* 26(7), 535–541.

Gitlin, L.N., Burgio L., Czaja S., Mahoney D., Gallagher-Thompson D., Burns R., et al. (2003) Effect of multi-component interventions on caregiver burden and depression: The REACH multi-site initiative at 6 months follow-up. *Psychology and Aging* 18, 361–374.

Hamilton, H.E. (1994) *Conversation with an Alzheimer's Patient. An Interactional Sociolinguistic Study*. Cambridge and New York: Cambridge University Press.

Hoeffer, B., Rader, J., Mckenzie, D., Lavelle, M., & Stewart, B. (1997) Reducing aggressive behavior during bathing cognitively impaired nursing home residents. *Journal of Gerontological Nursing* 23, 16–23.

Kagan, A., Black, S.E., Duchan, J.F., Simmons-Mackie, N., & Square, P. (2001) Training volunteers as conversation partners using "supported conversation for adults with aphasia" (SCA): Controlled trial. *Journal of Speech-Language-Hearing Research* 44(3), 624–638.

Lock, S., Wilkinson, R., & Bryan, K. (2008) *Supporting Partners of People with Aphasia in Relationships and Conversation*. Milton Keynes: Speechmark.

McCallion, P., Toseland, R.W., Lacey, D., & Banks, S. (1999) Educating nursing assistants to communicate more effectively with nursing home residents with dementia. *The Gerontologist* **39**, 546–558.

Murray, L.L. (1998) Longitudinal treatment of primary progressive aphasia: A case study. *Aphasiology* **12**(7), 651–672.

Murphy, J., Gray, C.M., & Cox, S. (2007) How 'Talking Mats' can help people with dementia to express themselves: Full report. Joseph Rowntree Foundation. Downloaded from: http://www.jrf.org.uk/sites/files/jrf/2128-talking-mats-dementia.pdf

National Collaborating Centre for Mental Health commissioned by the Social Care Institute for Excellence National Institute for Health and Clinical Excellence (revised 2011) The NICE-SCIE Guideline on Supporting People with Dementia and their Carers in Health and Social Welfare. National Clinical Practice Guideline Number 42 published by The British Psychological Society and Gaskell. Downloaded from: http://www.nice.org.uk/nicemedia/live/10998/30320/30320.pdf

Perkins, L. Whitworth, A., & Lesser, R. (1998) Conversing in dementia: A conversation analytic approach. *Journal of Neurolinguistics* **12**(1–2), 35–53.

Ripich, D., Ziol, E., & Lee, M.M. (1998) Longitudinal effects of communication training on caregivers of persons with Alzheimer's disease. *Clinical Gerentologist* **19**(2), 37–55.

Ripich, D., Ziol, E., Fritsch, T., & Durand, E.J. (1999) Training Alzheimer's disease caregivers for successful communication. *Clinical Gerentologist* **21**(1), 37–56.

Rogers, J.C., Holm, M.B., Burgio, L.D., Hsu, C., Hardon, M., & McDowell, B.J. (2000) Excess disability during morning care in nursing home residents with dementia. *International Psychogeratrics* **12**(2), 267–282.

Royal College of Speech and Language Therapists (2005) Speech and language therapy provision for people with dementia. RCSLT Position Paper. London: RCSLT. Downloaded from: www.rcslt.org/resources/publications

Royal College of Speech and Language Therapists (2009) Resource manual for commissioning and planning services for SLCN dementia. Downloaded from: www.rcslt.org/resources/publications

Small, J.A. & Gutman, G. (2002). Recommended and reported use of communication strategies in Alzheimer caregiving. *Alzheimer Disease and Associated Disorders* **16**(4) 270-278.

Smith, M. & Buckwater, K. (2005) Behaviours associated with dementia. *American Journal of Nursing* **105**(7), 40–52.

Taylor, C., Kingma, R.M., Croot, K., & Nickels, L. (2009) Speech pathology services for primary progressive aphasia: Exploring and emerging area of practice. *Aphasiology* **23**(2), 161–174.

Tonkovich, J.D. (1999) Managing the long-term communication and memory consequences of dementia. *Neurophysiology and Neurogenic Speech and Language Newsletter* **9**(5), 9–14.

Volkmer, A. (2006) Counseling and aphasia: A multidisciplinary approach to families. *Bulletin* I, 649.

Wong, S.B., Anand, R., Chapman, S.B., Rackley, A., & Zientz, J. (2009) When nouns and verbs degrade: Facilitating communication in semantic dementia. *Aphasiology* **23**(2), 286–301.

7 Decision making and capacity in dementia: Our role as speech and language therapists

Allied health professionals are often apprehensive and lack confidence in assessing mental capacity. In the UK, this feeling may have increased as a consequence of the 2005 Mental Health Capacity Act. Skinner, Joiner, Chesters et al. (2010) suggest that clinicians feel worried that they do not have the experience, knowledge, training or skills and that such an assessment should be the role of a specialist such as a psychologist or psychiatrist. The authors emphasize, however, that capacity assessment is not a specialist skill. Health professionals such as speech and language therapists should feel confident in this area, as they may be one of the most appropriately skilled team members to conduct such an assessment.

This chapter will update you on some of the legislation surrounding capacity assessment for people with dementia, as well as providing some practical guidance on assessing capacity for different types of decisions. Finally, we highlight some examples of how these approaches can be linked to the research literature. We also discuss how speech and language therapists may be involved in supporting patients and preparing them for when decision making becomes a problem.

Introduction to capacity assessments

The Mental Capacity Act states:

> "...a person lacks capacity in relation to a matter if at the material time he is unable to make a decision for himself in relation to the matter because of an impairment of, or a disturbance in the functioning of, the mind or brain."
> (Department of Health, 2005)

An individual is assumed to have capacity until it has been demonstrated that they do not. There are a number of important documents and guidelines to support us in the process of conducting capacity assessments, the most important of which is the Mental Capacity Act (2005). This was designed to provide clarification on what it means to lack capacity and to support professionals in the complex area of capacity assessment as well as any recommendations that may be made by the team as a consequence of their assessments (see Table 7.1 for further practical guidance for capacity assessment). The NICE guidelines for dementia (updated in 2011) make a number of clear recommendations about the role of health professionals in regard to capacity and decision making with people with dementia. This is also a valuable document to support and clarify our role, covering aspects such as consent to treatment, advance statements, lasting power of attorney and decision making about future care choices.

In the past, assessing capacity has been dominated by medical staff or psychologists. It is, however, increasingly recognized that other members of the multidisciplinary team have the expertise to support this process. Assessing a patient's capacity to make decisions is becoming a standard part of our role as speech and language therapists. Most often, these are decisions related to a patient's medical care, their finances and their discharge from hospital or admission to residential facilities. Often we will be called upon not only to assess the patient's ability (or capacity) to make these decisions but also to make recommendations for how to best support the individual in conversations related to these decisions, such as recommending the use of particular prompts or pictures.

Table 7.1 Summary of key practical points for capacity assessment.

Key points when assessing capacity to make a decision (from the Mental Health Act, 2005)
A lack of capacity cannot be established merely by reference to:
(a) a person's age or appearance, or
(b) a condition he has, or
(c) an aspect of his behaviour.
A person is unable to make a decision for himself if he is unable to:
(a) understand the information relevant to the decision
(b) retain that information
(c) use or weigh that information as part of the process of making the decision, or
(d) communicate his decision (whether by talking, using sign language or any other means).
A person is not to be regarded as unable to understand the information relevant to a decision if he is able to understand an explanation of it given to him in a way that is appropriate to his circumstances (using simple language, visual aids or any other means).
The fact that a person is able to retain the information relevant to a decision for a short period only does not prevent him from being regarded as able to make the decision.

A brief history of capacity and decision making in health care

The area of capacity assessment is influenced by two core ethical principles: firstly, respect for liberty and autonomy of the individual and, secondly, protection of the vulnerable individual (Moye & Marson, 2007). Respect for autonomy is considered a key principle in health care (Beauchamp & Childress, 2001). Yet the responsibility that clinicians have to protect people from harm can, at times, directly conflict with respecting a person's liberty to make bad decisions. It can be very difficult to balance these two factors when assessing decision-making capacity (Lo, 1990).

In the earlier part of the 20th century, capacity was decided purely on the basis of a medical diagnosis. Patients were also deemed to entirely lack capacity in global terms, whilst now it is viewed as more appropriate to consider capacity as specific to different situations (Lo, 1990). There has also been a shift to a more intricate understanding of key functional abilities required for different decision-making domains and risks surrounding different types of decisions.

Capacity in the health setting refers to the judgement of the clinician as to whether a person can perform a specific task or make specific decisions. Such decisions about capacity are ultimately legal judgements, which are then enforced by law. Moye and Marson (2007) highlight eight major areas that can be considered relevant to older adults with dementia or other neuropsychiatric illnesses. These include decision making related to financial capacity, independent living, treatment consent, testamentary capacity, research consent, sexual consent, voting and driving.

This division into different areas of decision making has resulted in many attempts to develop specific risk assessments and standardized assessment tools to measure whether people have capacity in these areas. Most of these assessment tools try to improve and support the notoriously low reliability of general clinical decision making by focusing on relevant skills required for these tasks (Moye & Marson, 2007). Moye, Karel, Azar and Guerrers (2004) also highlight that this is incredibly difficult as there is no accepted standard criterion for capacity that can allow validity of different tools to be compared to one another. Other tools have attempted to balance risks and identify levels of capacity required. Lo (1990) emphasizes that this can give clinicians too much control over individuals who disagree with them, rather than considering the patient's perspective and judging what the patient would consider a risk.

Importantly, adults are generally presumed to be competent unless a court of law or a health care professional identifies that an individual's ability to make a decision is questionable (Lo, 1990); this is the 'presumption of capacity' (Bellhouse, Holland, Clare & Gunn, 2001). Questions about an individual's capacity tend to be raised when that person has demonstrated cognitive or psychiatric difficulties that might affect their ability to understand, evaluate and articulate decisions (Moye, Karel, Azar & Gurrera, 2004). What can be particularly tricky is that these are probably individuals who have previously been managing areas such as finances quite competently (Moye et al., 2004). What is additionally complex when assessing people with a progressive disease such as dementia is judging at what point the condition affects the skill of decision making such that the individual is deemed no longer competent to make their own decisions.

Moye et al. (2004) highlight that this area of capacity assessment has developed an increasingly more important profile as part of routine clinical practice with patients with dementia. They attribute this to the increase in the numbers of adults surviving to older age and consequently the increased incidence of dementia. They also highlight the changes in culture and finances over the last century, which have resulted in families living further away from one another. This may leave older adults more vulnerable to exploitation from strangers. Moye et al. (2004) also highlight the impact that increases in wealth in families in Western societies have had, resulting in increased concerns around financial vulnerability.

If an individual is deemed to lack capacity in an area, they may require an individual, such as a guardian or power of attorney, to act on their behalf. In some cases, an individual may have already been legally appointed and will only act once the patient is deemed to have no capacity. In most cases, there will probably already be someone acting in this role, albeit informally. As part of the process of capacity assessment it may be important to recommend that this role is legally recognized in order to protect all parties involved from future litigation.

Who is involved in assessing a patient's capacity?

In short, any member of the clinical team could be involved in assessing a person's capacity in the healthcare setting. Capacity assessment is a complicated process that requires expertise from across disciplines of health and law (Moye et al., 2004). Up until now, the literature on capacity assessment has focused on medical issues such as treatment consent, do not resuscitate orders and withdrawing or withholding life-sustaining treatment (Kirschner, Stocking, Wagner, Foye & Siegler, 2001). Increasingly, however, research highlights capacity issues arising in less acute environments. This includes areas such as rehabilitation services where informed consent, and decisions related to discharge, as well as refusal of recommendations have been highlighted as concerning capacity issues (Kirschner et al., 2001).

Seeking advice from colleagues is considered good practice in the field of capacity assessment (Bellhouse et al., 2001) and many clinicians will carry out joint assessments, or get a second opinion as required. Some clinicians will advocate using formal assessment measures; however, standard mental status screens such as a Mini Mental State Examination (MMSE) are not considered "accurate or acceptable predictors of decisional capacity" (Moye et al., 2007). As Moye et al. (2007) explain, patients may fail these tests yet be competent to make specific decisions about health care or finances.

Dreer, Devivo, Novack and Marson (2012) describe impaired decisional capacity as a significant challenge for clinicians, who must frequently determine if a person has decisional capacity to resume independent decision making. This often requires a multidisciplinary approach where clinicians who are most able to inform the particular decision-making area may be better employed for different assessments. The occupational therapist or social worker may be well placed to advise on finances based on their knowledge of the patient's skills and funds, whereas the medical team is probably best placed to discuss consent for the specific medical procedures they have recommended. Speech and language therapists are likely to be involved in any one of the assessments. Bellhouse et al. (2001) and Bourgeois and Hickey (2009) emphasize that the advice and skills of a speech and language therapist can assist a capacity assessment. The Royal College of Speech and Language Therapists (2005) clearly states that speech and language therapists "are uniquely qualified to assess an individual's capacity to communicate and understand information". The RCSLT also recommends that speech and language therapists should provide advice on how to present information to support patients for whom communication impairment may prevent them from being able to make a 'free choice'. This could include using carefully-chosen pictures, verbal and non-verbal communication, giving people opportunities to talk in indirect ways and giving people time to express themselves (Murphy, Oliver & Cox, 2010).

Flew and Holly (2011) advocate that speech and language therapists have a number of different roles to play in assessing a person's capacity. They highlight that we can act as educator and advisor to the person carrying out the assessment, or act to engage and support the person being assessed to enable them to participate to their best possible level in the assessment. Yet, equally, they suggest we can participate as an assessor. Finally, we may also act as the implementer following assessment, addressing areas of need or change that have been identified during the assessment process. Flew and Holly (2011) warn that, although taking on the role of assessor is a vital part of our role as clinicians, it can have a negative effect on the therapeutic relationship, and can be extremely time consuming. Having said this, it is worth referring back to the recommendation previously made: to conduct such an assessment alongside a colleague. This can assist in balancing this interplay of roles and reducing the risk of a negative impact on the therapeutic roles.

Assessing capacity to consent to medical treatment

Assessing an individual's ability to consent to medical treatment is considered particularly important due to the significant risks to an individual's health and wellbeing. If the wrong decision is made, in the worst scenario this may result in unintended severe illness or death. Speech and language therapists can have a significant impact on this process as maximizing an individual's comprehension can aid them in weighing up their decision appropriately, and enabling them to express their opinion will support a more mutually positive outcome.

Moye et al. (2007) describe consent capacity as "a patient's cognitive and emotional capacity to select among treatment alternatives or to refuse treatment". These authors suggest that informed consent is more distinctive from other types of capacity decisions as it arises in medical rather than legal settings and generally involves health professionals rather than lawyers. Perhaps health professionals are therefore somewhat more familiar and comfortable with this type of assessment. In fact, we are constantly assessing consent of patients to participate in therapy sessions. Consent is not solely an issue as regards medical procedures. Decisions about whether to go out or participate in an activity or whether to accept extra home or respite care are all aspects of life to which the person with dementia may or may not wish to consent (Cameron & Murphy, 2006). The NICE dementia guidelines (updated, 2011) advocate for this ongoing process of checking consent, stating that:

> "Health and social care professionals should always seek valid consent from people with dementia. This should entail informing the person of options, and checking that he or she understands, that there is no coercion and that he or she continues to consent over time. If the person lacks the capacity to make a decision, the provisions of the Mental Capacity Act 2005 must be followed."

As previously mentioned, the UK Mental Capacity Act (2005) emphasizes four core abilities required to make a consensual decision. These are the ability to:

- express a decision or choice
- understand information related to the decision, i.e. attend to what is said and encode this information
- appreciate or weigh up the information and risks related to this decision, requiring insight, foresight and judgement, and finally,
- reason and compare different alternatives through analyzing and comparing information.

This seemingly straightforward process can be fraught with minefields. It can be particularly difficult to ensure people understand the impact of their decision yet avoid coercing patients when explaining the relevant issues. This is particularly difficult when asking someone to consent to participate in research (Cameron & Murphy, 2006).

The other, perhaps more clinically relevant tension, is the obligation to respect unconventional choices, but protect people from harm. Therefore, enhancing the individual's ability to make decisions is vital through the use of strategies such as speaking slowly, not raising your voice, facing the person, giving them time, using communication aids, inviting in familiar people to support the process, repeating the discussion and allowing decisions to be considered in the person's own time. Even postponing the decision until other issues that may be confounding a person's capacity can be treated can be time efficient. Using questions that ask the individual to paraphrase a statement, summarize a discussion, explain the pros and cons of a procedure and asking them about the consequences, are some examples of appropriate questions that might be used in this type of conversation (Lo, 1990). Lo (1990) highlights that good listening and interview skills as well as negotiation are essential to capacity assessments, and although seemingly time intensive, can reduce the need for more time if patients refuse treatments. Murphy, Gray and Cox (2007) also found that, at each session, consent needed to be revisited because participants had forgotten previous discussions. This highlights the need for clinicians to revisit consent to participate in therapy sessions at each new session.

A person's capacity to make medical decisions is unique in some ways when compared to other types of capacity, in that it cannot be challenged unless a patient refuses treatment that the team feels may be beneficial to them (Lo, 1990; Bellhouse et al., 2001). In fact, the dilemma here is that, even if that individual lacks capacity to make a decision and is refusing treatment, it can be very difficult to continue giving treatment if, for example, they are physically resisting a treatment or refusing to participate in a therapy session. This is where a decision made in that individual's best interest may still need to incorporate their wishes and those of their family and evidence of what would be consistent with their beliefs. For example, if someone has previously frequently declined treatments, it may not be out of character for them to refuse this treatment. So some treatments will require both consent and capacity. But the decision in this case rests with the treating doctor or other health professional. This is perhaps a familiar concept to speech and language therapists when patients refuse dysphagia management recommendations such as thickened drinks. Even if they do not have capacity to understand the risks surrounding this decision it is difficult to enforce the recommendations without the patient's consent as they can often simply refuse to drink. So, in these cases, it is not uncommon that patients will continue with thin fluids even though there may be a risk associated.

Importantly, Bellhouse et al. (2001) remind us that capacitous consent to treatment must also be informed and therefore the individual assessing the patient's capacity requires the knowledge of the procedure, including the benefit and risks. This means the person doing the capacity assessment will therefore likely also be the individual who will be responsible for the treatment or procedure. So although speech and language therapists may be involved in assessing an individual's skills to consent to a medical procedure or intervention, it is most likely that we will be acting in a role that supports the person with dementia to be able to make a decision in these cases. That is, we will be advising team members and colleagues about the best way to present information to a person with dementia in order to allow them to make an informed decision. This is an important difference compared to other types of capacity assessments. Table 7.2 (see p.185) provides a list of example questions for assessing decision-making abilities related to consent.

Case Study 1: Mrs H

Mrs H is a 98-year-old lady who lives at home with her daughter, who is also her main carer. Mrs H is deaf and partially sighted, she has severe arthritis and is unable to mobilize easily, using a four-wheel frame with supervision around her home and a wheelchair outdoors. She has moderate vascular dementia, and has recently had a stroke that has left her with swallowing difficulties. In hospital, she had been advised to take thickener in all her drinks, which she had done, but on going home she started to refuse these. On assessment, she continued to present with difficulties tolerating thin fluids. The speech and language therapist provided an explanation of the swallow function using a simple diagram to highlight what can happen when fluids get into the lungs and emphasized the risk of chest infections, as well as the pros and cons of thickening fluids. Mrs H reported that she understood this risk, but that she felt she enjoyed her cups of tea too much to continue using thickener. She stated that she had not had any chest infections to date, and that if she did that this would be OK as she was getting older, but she might reconsider it then. Mrs H's daughter confirmed that Mrs H had not had a chest infection to date and that these statements were consistent with her previous decision to stop taking thickener following her first stroke approximately ten years earlier (before she had shown any signs of cognitive deterioration or been diagnosed with dementia). The therapist liaised with Mrs H's GP, who attended a home visit with the therapist. Mrs H was unable to recall meeting the speech and language therapist before, but was able to recall the risks of fluids going down the wrong way when presented with the diagram and asked open questions, and provided the same rationale as at the previous visit. Both clinicians felt that the patient was making an informed decision consistent with her beliefs. The speech and language therapist continued to monitor Mrs H via one further visit and a follow-up telephone call. Consequently, Mrs H's daughter was given the speech and language therapist's contact details and advised to contact her should Mrs H experience any further difficulties or should she have any more concerns. Mrs H was readmitted to hospital one year later with another stroke, having managed without any chest infections over that period.

What does the research say about decision-making capacity in dementia?

There are a small number of articles where researchers have attempted to decipher what aspects of capacity are affected in people with dementia. They have focused very much on consent capacity and on the differences between different stages of dementia. There is general agreement amongst researchers and clinicians that these skills decline as the disease progresses (Moye et al., 2007) and that people with dementia may have some capacity in the mild stage, but that this should be individually assessed. The other point, which is debated in the literature, is the method of assessing consent capacity. There is general agreement that formal assessment tools are not necessarily better than structured interviews. The following provides a summary of these studies.

The research tells us that the consent capacity of individuals with dementia compared to individuals without dementia is severely reduced. This is due to difficulties in the areas of understanding, but also reasoning and appreciation report Marson, Cody et al. (1995, cited by Moye et al., 2007). The same authors cite research by Marson, Annis, McInturf, Bartolucci and Harell (1999) who found that people with mild Alzheimer's disease had difficulties answering questions, and frequently became confused and were unable to consider the theoretical examples given in consent capacity assessments. Moye et al. (2004) conducted a study to examine how adults with mild and moderate dementia compared to healthy control group adults on decision making around consent capacity. The participants presented with a mixture of different dementia types. The researchers used three different formal tools with the participants that were designed to assess capacity to make medical decisions: the MacArthur Competence Assessment Tool for Treatment; the Hopemont Capacity Assessment Interview; and the Capacity to Consent Instrument. These tools used specific questions to elicit the patients' understanding of the hypothesized treatment, asked them why they were having the treatment, why they were making the choice to have the treatment, and finally rated whether or not they clearly expressed a decision. The study showed that all patients with dementia performed less well than people without dementia on measures of understanding, although patients with mild dementia generally performed within the range of normal. It also revealed that the different measures assessed appreciation very differently, resulting in most people with dementia passing this on one test and on another test many of the control group failing. Similarly, the different measures were inconsistent in their rating of reasoning across both the control and dementia groups. Finally, the study found that all participants with mild and moderate dementia were able to express a decision or choice on all measures. Moye et al. (2004) concluded that assessment tools should be interpreted with a focus on individual situations and be facilitated by use of strategies to compensate for impairments. They highlight that clinical situations are often not structured strictly as formal evaluations so the use of notes, diagrams and references is common, similarly the use of communication aids to facilitate comprehension for aphasic people will be common.

Perhaps one of the most concerning findings from the literature is that it is not only formal assessments that demonstrate reduced reliability across tools, but also that clinicians completing informal structured interviews to assess consent capacity demonstrate little agreement on whether patients had capacity or not (Marson, McInturff, et al., 1995 cited by Moye et al., 2007). Moye et al. (2007) attribute this to the fact that measurement strategies developed for one patient may work less well with other patients. They summarize a number of studies that examine the association between capacity measures and cognitive measures for different conditions. They found that different factors predicted difficulties on different tasks, so, for example, patients with Alzheimer's dementia who had difficulties with conceptualization, verbal fluency and naming demonstrated difficulties in understanding, appreciating and reasoning related to a medical decision. On the other hand, patients with Parkinson's dementia who had executive difficulties and memory impairments demonstrated most difficulties in understanding and reasoning related to a decision. However, the authors emphasize that, with training clinicians can demonstrate increased reliability. Moye et al. (2007) also reflect on the different skills that different clinicians bring to capacity assessments and urge that these different approaches need to be explored.

However, we can learn from other client groups in this respect. Skinner et al. (2010) published an article on assessing the treatment consent capacity of adults with learning difficulties. The authors were part of a multidisciplinary team (Capacity Assessment Team) who set up a service model for assessing the consent capacity of adults with learning difficulties referred to ophthalmology for intervention. They describe setting up a screening system which considered individuals' communication skills, their mental health status and understanding of the decision using an initial accessible leaflet. They also report using a full assessment, which included open questions, contextual discussions of recent hospital admissions, semi-structured interviewing techniques and vignettes once patients had passed the initial screening phase. If the patient failed the initial screening phase, the medical team were advised of this and recommendations made to proceed in the patient's best interests. In this case, the team would offer to support this best interest decision. If the patient demonstrated capacity the individual would be supported to attend their medical appointment, where the consent would be confirmed by the medical team using the appropriately developed supports (e.g. picture cards). Figure 7.1 outlines the decision-making flow chart used by the team.

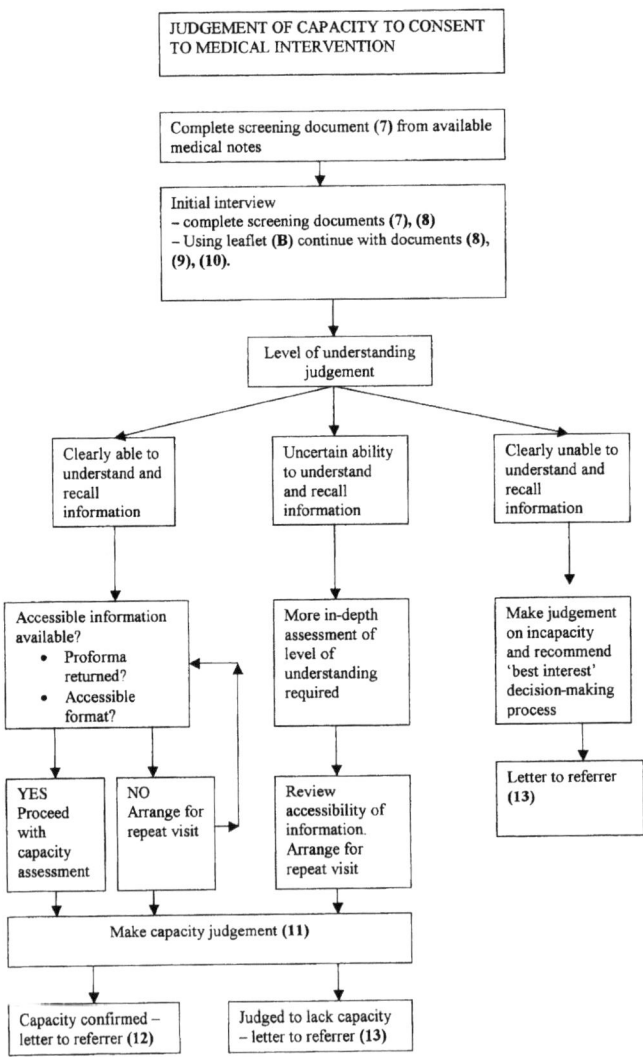

Figure 7.1 The decision-making flowchart when judging capacity to consent to medical interventions designed and used by the capacity assessment team (Skinner et al., 2010).

Decision-making capacity to manage finances

Assessing an individual's decision-making capacity to manage their own finances is considered particularly important because of the significant risks to an individual's wellbeing. If the patient makes the wrong decisions they may be left vulnerable to unpaid bills, debt build up and bankruptcy, as well as increased vulnerability to scams. The speech and language therapist can have a significant role in this process, both as an assessor and facilitator, although we are more likely to be called upon as an assessor of financial capacity. This will involve assessing the reading and writing skills required to support financial management, as well as evaluating the verbal communication and problem-solving skills involved in managing financial transactions. The speech and language therapist may also be involved in supporting the individual to understand the rationale for the assessment, and enable them to express preferences about who they would like to support them in managing their finances in the future should they be found to lack capacity in this area.

The capacity to manage financial affairs is considered a fundamental instrumental activity of daily living "critical to independent functioning of adults in our society" (Marson, Stephen, Sawrie, Snyder, et al., 2000). Marson et al. also emphasize that it is "possibly the best single litmus for capacity to live independently". Moye et al. (2007) describe financial capacity as "a broad range of conceptual, pragmatic and judgment abilities". This includes skills ranging from counting and checking coins and cash and using a cash point and writing cheques, as well as checking and managing bank statements and bills, writing a will and deciding on financial investments. Finances are a particularly complex skill that will be different for each individual, depending on his or her social and financial situation.

Dreer et al. (2012) highlight that impairment in mental and written arithmetic, reduced semantic financial knowledge, poor self-awareness, insight, impulsivity, disinhibition and short-term memory difficulties can all negatively influence financial decision making. Financial capacity requires three particular types of knowledge and skills:

- declarative knowledge, which is the ability to describe information related to financial activities such as knowing how much money is paid into one's account every month from one's wage or benefits
- the procedural knowledge required to carry out financially-related tasks such as writing a cheque

- judgement; the skill of making appropriate decisions to protect one's financial interests (Marson et al., 2000).

This range of skills can be considered a spectrum, where one individual may be able to manage small amounts of monies, e.g. once given some cash they are able to go to the shops and purchase a small number of items, also checking their change appropriately. This person may only need support for bigger financial tasks such as managing their accounts and paying bills. In comparison, a different person may require more assistance to manage all aspects of their monies. If an individual does need support, it is important to engage them in conversation to identity whom they would prefer to provide them with the required support. This is a key area of financial capacity assessment as it can not only reveal their level of insight but also provide them with the opportunity for choice and support. This is where it is key to ensure a patient with a communication impairment is able to express a preference if possible, as patients are more likely to consent and comply with recommendations if they have been able to voice a choice.

It is worth mentioning the literature on financial capacity in adults with dementia, even though it is sparse and only recently emerging. There is evidence from assessments of adults with mild Alzheimer's dementia that they will have difficulties in both simple and more complex financial tasks and, perhaps more concerningly, a lack of insight to this difficulty (Moye et al., 2007). There is also evidence that people with Mild Cognitive Impairment (MCI) will start to demonstrate difficulties in these areas compared to healthy adults of the same age (Griffith, Belue, Sicola, Kryzywanski, et al., 2003). This is important as it is generally assumed that people with MCI are able to manage much more independently than people with dementia, yet evidence shows they are already becoming vulnerable in this area of daily life. Table 7.2 provides a list of example questions for assessing financial capacity.

Case study 2: Mr I

Mr I was in his mid 50s. He lived at home with his wife and three teenage children prior to his admission to the assessment ward with suspected frontotemporal dementia on the background of a brain injury sustained after falling down the stairs of his home three years previously. Mrs I reported that over the past two months Mr I had become increasingly aggressive and suspicious. He had threatened her and on one occasion had also threatened their son. She also reported that he appeared to forget things more often, and had recently got lost on a few occasions on the way home from the shops he goes to every week. She reported that prior to Mr I's brain injury he had managed all their finances, but that since his injury she had taken over this responsibility as his deputy. She reported that recently he had hidden a number of bills and statements before she had been able to get to the post, and had become very frustrated and agitated when she refused to allow him to apply for credit cards. Mrs I stated that this was an area which was causing increasing concern (among other concerns); although she wished him to return home, she felt he couldn't return to managing the finances but was unsure how to communicate this to him. During his admission the occupational therapist (OT), psychologist and speech and language therapist reviewed Mr I's ability to manage his finances. This involved:

- Liaising with Mrs I about the family banking (including bank account held, benefit details, etc), managing small change at the shops and discussing how Mr I had managed these prior to his injury (was he frugal, or often in debt?)
- Asking Mr I about his knowledge of the family assets and income, etc
- Asking him to participate in functional assessment with the OT using a small amount of money at the shops
- Assessing his ability to read a bill and identify important information relevant to payment, and checking information was accurate
- Asking Mr I to explain his rationale for applying for two credit cards and why he supposed his wife was unhappy about this, also discussing the benefits and disadvantages to having a credit card
- Asking him how he would manage if he ran into difficulties, using vignette examples of what could go wrong.

Assessment indicated that Mr I continued to lack capacity to manage his and the family's finances, although he was able to manage small amounts of money when going to the shops to buy a small number of items. He was unable to attend to the task and demonstrated reduced attention in reading a bill to check information as accurate. Mr I was also unable to weigh up the risks around applying for a credit card, or make any plan as to how he would make repayments. However, the team felt it would be useful for his wife to be able to involve him in the task of managing the bills, as it had previously been part of his role. Together with Mrs I, the team devised a structured method whereby Mr I was able to sit with his wife reading out bill information whilst she completed the banking tasks and reported on what she was doing. Mr and Mrs I reported ongoing satisfaction in this task six months after discharge.

Decision-making capacity to decide on living situation

An individual's decision-making capacity to decide on their discharge destination or ability to live independently is considered particularly important due to the significant risks to their physical health. There are also risks to their social wellbeing to consider. If the patient makes the wrong decisions here it could result in them not being able to manage basic care tasks such as taking medications and feeding themselves (self-neglect). It can also have implications for managing highly risky situations, for example if there was a fire in their home, that could ultimately lead to death or serious illness. Speech and language therapists can have a significant impact on this assessment process, again as both assessors and facilitators.

This is a vast area of functioning; it can cover almost all aspects of daily living skills including basic daily care such as washing, personal hygiene and dressing, but also cooking, buying food and keeping the home clean and habitable. There are also more complex things to consider, such as ability and safety awareness in the local community, cognition and navigation around the community as well as problem-solving skills such as the ability to call for help when needed. Moye et al. (2007) highlight that this area of need is often unrecognized and misunderstood, particularly when considering risks such as neglect and withdrawal from services.

This is again an area where the speech and language therapist can act as both assessor and facilitator. Indeed, assessing an individual's ability to communicate on the phone in a potential emergency, speak to shop assistants to get what they need, and communicate to local care providers such as their GP about how they are managing could be key parts of the assessment process. As with consent capacity, the speech and language therapist can have an important role in supporting a patient to understand the options available to them and make an informed decision about where they would like to live. It is also vital that the patient is afforded the option of highlighting where he or she would prefer to live. Table 7.2 provides a list of example questions for assessing decision-making abilities related to discharge.

As previously discussed in reference to consent capacity, it can be difficult to enforce a decision made by someone other than the patient if the patient doesn't consent to a specific living situation. And although there are ways of supporting this (such as locked environments), it can be quite difficult to maintain this environment and can impact significantly on an individual's wellbeing. This option must be carefully considered. The Deprivation of Liberty Safeguards (DoLS) were introduced in 2007 as part of the Mental Capacity Act (2005). DoLS apply to people suffering from a 'mental disorder or disability of the mind', such as dementia, who lack the capacity to give informed consent for the arrangements made for their care and or treatment. In these cases, it may be that depriving them of their liberty is necessary and in their best interests in order to protect them from harm. The safeguards cover patients in hospitals and people in care homes. DoLS are designed to protect the interests of a person, to ensure that they are given the care they need in the least restrictive environment, so preventing them from being deprived of their liberty. It may be that the team decides to apply for a DoLS in the event the person, or the person's family, object to their admission to hospital or their transfer to a residential setting.

Case study 3: Mr J

Mr J was a man in his late 50s who contracted HIV some years ago, He had been living alone in the community until recently but had not been taking his medications. This had led to a deterioration in his health and admission to hospital. He had continued to deteriorate in hospital, refusing medications and becoming increasingly unmanageable. Mr J was transferred from a local hospital where they were struggling to manage his increasingly aggressive behaviour and agitation. He was admitted to specialist care and sectioned as it was felt he was psychotic. He also presented with significant cognitive and communication difficulties. During the course of his admission he started to take his medication again and, as he became more well, his cognition and communication improved somewhat. On imaging, however, it was felt that he presented with white matter changes consistent with HIV dementia. On making plans for his consequent discharge from the unit, a home visit was conducted to his home. This visit highlighted that his home was not safe to be lived in. The team also felt that Mr J's physical and cognitive difficulties meant that he would require 24-hour support and supervision. During the course of his admission, Mr J expressed a desire to return to his home. His brothers were located but reported they had been unaware of his admission, and also that Mr J had always lived in what would be considered unsanitary conditions. On discussion around discharge, they stated that they would be unable to provide the support he required, as did the local mental and disability services.

The speech and language therapist and psychologist conducted an initial capacity assessment, using a structured interview model, to examine Mr J's ability to make decisions related to discharge. On assessment, Mr J insisted that he wished to return home, and that he did not believe his physical or cognitive difficulties would prevent him from managing safely. He stated that he would likely discontinue taking his medications if he went home, but that this was OK as he did not feel they were helping. Mr J refused further discussion on this topic. At a later date the therapists returned to review this assessment. At this point, the clinicians explained the team's concern about his welfare and advised Mr J of what was being recommended, providing some written and pictoral information of residential homes in the area. It was also suggested that he could return to his home to visit and collect his belongings. Mr J stated that he understood the team were concerned about his welfare and agreed that he wanted to remain well, stating that the support from the staff at the unit would likely be helpful. He consented to the referral being made and was keen to visit his home. Although Mr J's feelings about the residential centre continued to fluctuate, he remained agreeable to this plan in further similar conversations using written and pictoral supports. Upon visiting his home to collect his belongings, he expressed surprise at the state of the house but insisted that he felt he could have lived there independently and that he was not unwell, although he understood the team's recommendations were around keeping him as well as possible.

The team agreed that Mr J lacked the capacity to make this decision. At this time it was felt his needs would be best met in the unit and he was later discharged to one of the residential units which he had expressed an interest in. During his admission to hospital Mr J has been detained under the mental health act but when this has revised on his discharge the team at the residential facility decided to apply for a Deprivation of Liberty Safeguard.

Table 7.2 Example questions for capacity assessment (this is not an exhaustive list by any means and just provides some ideas).

	Assessment questions (examples)
Consent capacity	Explain area of medical concern and recommended treatment Advise patient of alternatives to recommended treatment. Provide information on risks of treatment and risks of choosing alternatives
	Ask patient to recall/repeat/rephrase or summarize this information
	Ask patient what their preference is
	Ask patient to explain the reason for their preference
	Ask patient what they think are the pros and cons of treatment and/or the alternatives to the recommended treatment
Financial capacity	Can you tell me who you bank with and how much money you have in your accounts? Or how much goes in or out of your account on a regular basis?
	(Give patient coins/notes) Tell me which one is £1, £5, etc. If you are in a shop and you are buying a drink for X amount of money; what would you pay with and how much change would they give you? (Give patient change.) Is this the right change? What would you do if you were not given the right change?
	If you had a budget of X for one month what would you spend it on?
	(Give patient a bill.) Can you tell me how much the outstanding amount is? Are there any errors on the bill? (Give blank cheque.) Can you fill out a cheque?
	(Consult with OT.) Can patient use cash point, e.g. read words on the screen and press correct buttons/talk to cashiers, with aid if appropriate?
	What are the risks of not checking your bank statement regularly? What are the risks of not checking your change in a shop? What are the risks of not paying off your credit card? What are the risks of not paying your bill on time?
	What would you do if you lost your bank card/you noticed an error on your statement?
	Who could you ask for help?
	What are the risks of making purchases on the internet?
	Why do you think these things would be difficult for you?
	Why do you think the team is concerned?
	Explain the team's concerns and recommendations and ask: Why do you think the team has recommended this?

(Continued overleaf)

Capacity to decide on discharge destination	What could be difficult when you go home?
	What do you have help with here in hospital?
	Who could you ask to help you?
	What are the risks of living on your own?
	What would happen if there were a fire/burglary, etc? (Ask patient to role play this if necessary.)
	(Consult with OT) Could you cook and clean for yourself independently? Could you get to the shops on your own?"
	What would you do if you fell over? (Consult with OT/PT.) What are the risks of falls in home? Can you mobilize safely around home?
	List some of the team's concerns and ask: Why do you think these things might be difficult for you?
	Explain the team's concerns and recommendations and ask: Why do you think the team has recommended this?

NB: OT = occupational therapist; PT = physiotherapist

Assessing other areas of capacity and decision making

Moye et al. (2007) emphasize that other areas of decision making, such as testamentary capacity, sexual consent and voting capacity, have received very little attention in the health literature to date. Although these may not be areas that will commonly need to be addressed with people with dementia it is worth understanding that, as a speech and language therapist, you may be called upon to support a patient in these areas, or even to assess their ability to make such decisions. In these cases, it is worth returning to the literature to identify any more recent relevant articles, consulting literature from other client groups such as learning disability and brain injury, and talking to your colleagues, your patient and their significant others to gauge how best to support or assess a person's decision-making.

It is, however, worthwhile touching on one of these areas of capacity, which centres primarily around patients within the mental health sector. The 2007 Mental Health Act states that individuals may be detained for treatment or assessment for a mental disorder. These individuals also have the legal right to be informed of the section they are subject to, and how to appeal. Most people with dementia are likely to be detained under the Mental Capacity Act rather than the Mental Health Act, but some might be detained by this method. Henson, Gilbertson, Azzopardi and Pope (2012) recently highlighted that, in mental health settings, there is evidence that around 60% of patients will routinely appeal a section, yet in the brain injury setting they found that as few as 17% of patients under section appealed. There is no similar data on the older adult population but one could safely assume that there might be a similar pattern where people with dementia are not appealing. Henson et al. (2012) hypothesize that it is likely that many of these patients are not appealing because they do not understand information given to them, or lack the ability to communicate adequately to commence this process. This is where speech and language therapists may need to support clinicians who are advising patients of the section and their rights to ensure this is communicated in a supportive and appropriate manner. Henson et al. (2012) advocate for speech and language therapists to train colleagues in these skills and suggest the development of communication aids to support these conversations. However, it is also worth considering that this in turn can lead to questions of whether our patients have the capacity to make those decisions to appeal their section. If they do not, then should someone, such as a guardian or power of attorney, be sought to act in the patients' best interest and to be present when they are informed of their rights and pursue such appeals, as appropriate, on their behalf?

As a discipline, we should be considering our patients' rights to voice their opinions or preferences. In fact, it may be that part of our role in these other areas of decision making is to advocate for our patients' rights to vote or challenge their section. And assessing that person's ability to do this may be secondary to this.

What does the literature say about communication strategies and aids to support capacity assessments and decision making?

There is some research in which investigators have examined types of communication strategies that can support assessment of decision-making capacity. These studies have focused predominantly on consent capacity. In fact, the majority of the research in the area of communication supports for capacity is dominated by evidence for the use of Talking Mats to support the decision-making process, and some of this research has even focused specifically on patients with dementia.

Cameron and Murphy (2006) examined the use of a number of strategies to support the assessment of capacity and the consent process for people with learning difficulties. Their study included the use of repetition, pauses to support processing of information, frequent prompts to attend to the topic, and pictures with written short sentences to illustrate the different steps of the study. Cameron and Murphy (2006) observed the individuals they were working with for positive signs of consent such as engagement through body language and eye contact and positive verbal or non-verbal responses. Doubtful responses were considered lower levels of eye contact, ambivalence and evidence that individuals were agreeing too quickly (without full comprehension). The researchers also asked carers for confirmation that they agreed with the interpretation of these responses. When the researchers compared the participants' consent ability to their comprehension levels, they found that those with a functional comprehension level at three and four information-carrying words were all able to consent independently. At lesser levels, the individual often needed more support than that offered and was sometimes unable to consent.

Diener and Bischof-Rosario (2004) describe a case study of a gentleman with severe communication deficits following a stroke, and the implementation of augmentative-alternative communication (AAC) in supporting the investigation of whether he had capacity to decide on end-of-life decisions. The authors explain that AAC can include gesture systems, keyboards, word or picture books and boards, speech generating devices and communication partner techniques to support or compensate for a communication deficit. They highlight that there may be ethical dilemmas involved in supporting such decision making around end-of-life decisions. However, they also go on to suggest that the clinician's role is not to assess capacity in this instance but to find a means to allow the individual to participate in this process such as developing a reliable communication aid. They advocate that talking with a patient is the only way to determine if that patient has the ability to understand and make a decision in light of relevant information provided. This not only highlights the vital role that speech and language therapists have in assessing decision-making capacity but also the importance of approaching capacity assessments as a team.

Talking Mats is a low technology communication framework developed at the university of Stirling, in Scotland. It is a simple system of picture symbols that are placed on a textured mat in a particular order to allow people to discuss and indicate their views about various options (as described in Chapter 4). Murphy et al. (2010) describe using a scale and inviting individuals with dementia to place images related to a particular topic into this visual scale. For example, if the discussion is around support for daily living, the person can place pictorial images of different activities on a scale, rating them as 'Things I can do on my own, things I am unsure about, and things I need support with' (see Figure 7.2). This can then become the basis for discussion about decisions surrounding discharge that might otherwise be conducted under the assumption that the individual did not have the capacity to participate in this. The recommendation is that the clinician should take a photo of the completed mat as a record of the conversation, acting as a permanent record of the decision and also used as a memory prompt in future conversations.

Murphy et al. (2007; 2010) conducted research to examine how people at different stages of dementia felt about their lives, particularly the activities they participated in, the people around them, the environment and themselves using Talking Mats to support conversation. They found that patients produced more reliable information when using Talking Mats than with a structured verbal conversation, when information was compared to real life events. In fact, they found that patients with mild dementia were able to improve their ability to weigh up the pros and cons of their decision and that using Talking Mats could assist conversations into later stages of dementia. Murphy et al. (2007) emphasize that using Talking Mats can increase the length of time in which people with dementia play an active role in decision making related to their lives. Family members, who are often appointed as powers of attorney (requiring them to make complex financial and sometimes medical decisions) but also are carers must make daily decisions about all aspects of daily living. The Talking Mats tools are a reliable method of ensuring that decision makers are able to have a conversation where they can take into account the individual's views, and likely reduce both parties' anxiety surrounding certain decisions (Murphy et al., 2010).

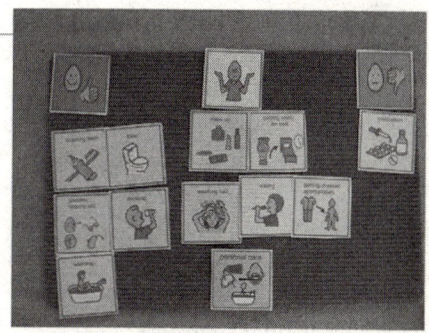

This Talking Mat shows..

How a person feels they are managing their personal care;

They feel quite confident they are managing their drinking, bathing, teeth etc.

There are some things they need help with like washing their hair, eating and dressing etc.

They are aware they are not managing their medication.

www.talkingmats.com

The JRF research project looked at how this framework could be used for both people with dementia and their carers to help both be involved in decision making

Figure 7.2 Example of how Talking Mats can be used to support people with dementia in expressing their decisions. (Reproduced by permission of J. Murphy, www.talkingmats.com)

In summary, using communication strategies and communication aids can increase a person's ability to demonstrate that they do have capacity to make certain decisions. This type of supported conversation can also ensure people are given an opportunity to express a preference or be informed of an event or procedure that will occur in the future. Lest we forget, the Mental Capacity Act states that the person making a decision in the patient's best interest if he is deemed to lack capacity "must, so far as reasonably practicable, permit and encourage the person to participate, or to improve his ability to participate, as fully as possible in any act done for him and any decision affecting him".

A word on moral dilemmas in capacity assessment

In years gone by, it was common practice to declare someone as entirely lacking in capacity to make any decisions. However, different situations are now considered to require different decision-making skills and are therefore assessed individually. It is important to ensure that the health professionals around the person do consider each type of decision separately so that these different areas of skill can be separately assessed and documented. To add to this complexity, an individual with dementia may demonstrate fluctuating capacity, where they lack capacity at one time yet not at another (Bellhouse et al., 2001). This is particularly tricky to manage and may involve specific recommendations around when they are most likely to be able to participate in decision-making conversations. Alternatively, it might be necessary to consider the suspension of a decision until that person regains their ability to participate.

Capacity assessments can be difficult and controversial at the best of times. Furthermore, these assessments will always be influenced by the clinician's personal beliefs, morals and values regarding how much protection should be given and the decision outcome itself (Lo, 1990). It is important to bear in mind that patients who make what we would consider unwise decisions may still have the capacity and the right to do so, even if we as health professionals disagree with their decisions (Bellhouse et al., 2001; Moye et al., 2007). It is our duty as health professionals to respect the autonomy of an individual when making decisions. A good example of this is where an individual's religious or spiritual beliefs influence their decision. As a clinician, one must find a way to be comfortable with this, be it that you use your peers, your supervision sessions or a debriefing session following particularly complex patients to ensure you have the opportunity to debrief, discuss and clarify these feelings.

The opinions of people with dementia are "often overlooked and their rights to information and free expression are fragile" (Tyrell et al., 2006, cited by Murphy et al., 2010). It is our duty as speech and language therapists to advocate for patients to have this freedom of expression and freedom of decision making where possible.

So what do we do after the capacity assessment?

Once the outcome of a capacity assessment has been decided the assessors must make recommendations about what should follow. These recommendations are likely to include strategies to support specific future decision-making situations. In the case of consent capacity this might mean the team makes a statement, for example that the person has capacity to make decisions as long as information is also written and repeated a number of times. These recommendations may then be passed to the medical professional conducting the procedure. Similar recommendations may be made for people who lack capacity. In this case, recommendations will be passed on to the individual who has been appointed in the role of lasting power of attorney or deputy as well as the medical professional conducting the procedure. However, it is also the team's responsibility to recommend the appointment of such an individual; a deputy, should the person with dementia lack capacity and not already have appointed anyone to such a position. If the position is not filled it requires that the family apply for position of deputy via the Court of Protection, with the support and advice of a solicitor.

The Mental Capacity Act (2005) describes the role of lasting power of attorney and deputy:

> "A lasting power of attorney is a power of attorney under which the donor ("P") confers on the donee (or donees) authority to make decisions about all or any of the following—
>
> P's personal welfare or specified matters concerning P's personal welfare, and
>
> P's property and affairs or specified matters concerning P's property and affairs,

and which includes authority to make such decisions in circumstances where P no longer has capacity."

"Appointing a deputy by the court of protection. This section applies if a person ("P") lacks capacity in relation to a matter or matters concerning—

P's personal welfare, or

P's property and affairs.

The court may—

by making an order, make the decision or decisions on P's behalf in relation to the matter or matters, or

appoint a person (a "deputy") to make decisions on P's behalf in relation to the matter or matters."

Should a person not have any family available to support them then an independent mental capacity advocate (IMCA) may be appointed. The Mental Capacity Act describes the IMCA's role to support the person in participating in decision making as much as possible. This may involve evaluating information, ascertaining what the person's preferences would be if they had capacity and asking for further medical opinions if required. The speech and language therapist has an important role in advising and guiding the IMCA in strategies to communicate with the person with dementia.

Supporting patients to plan in advance

"In an ideal world everyone would prepare an advance directive document specifying treatment preferences for a variety of medical conditions and end of life care." Bourgeois & Hickey, 2009

Yet in reality people rarely think through all of these scenarios; in fact, it can be scary and confronting to do this. Bourgeois and Hickey (2009) cite a study by Bravos et al. (2003) who found it is predominantly older, white, well-educated individuals of higher socioeconomic status who do have these in place. In many other instances, people may have made informal plans or had discussions about their wishes with family and friends, but very few people have considered advance directives or assigning a power of attorney. Advance directives are a legal document outlining specific wishes related to medical care, and medical power of attorney allows a person to appoint a proxy to act on their behalf. An advance directive document and a power of attorney application need to be completed whilst an individual still has capacity as they cannot be submitted after that capacity is lost.

The Mental Capacity Act (2005) describes advance directives as:

> "Advance decision" means a decision made by a person ("P"), after he has reached 18 and when he has capacity to do so, that if—
>
> at a later time and in such circumstances as he may specify, a specified treatment is proposed to be carried out or continued by a person providing health care for him, and
>
> at that time he lacks capacity to consent to the carrying out or continuation of the treatment,
>
> the specified treatment is not to be carried out or continued.

A decision or statement complies with this subsection only if—

> it is in writing,
>
> it is signed by P or by another person in P's presence and by P's direction,
>
> the signature is made or acknowledged by P in the presence of a witness, and
>
> the witness signs."

Supporting patients to consider and write advance directives, as well as advising people about the process of appointing an enduring power of attorney should be part of their package of care. In fact, many organizations advocate that this should be the role of the health professionals involved in dementia care.

The NICE dementia guidelines (2011) state that:

> "Health and social care professionals should discuss with the person with dementia, while he or she still has capacity, and his or her carer the use of:
>
> – advance statements (which allow people to state what is to be done if they should subsequently lose the capacity to decide or to communicate) advance decisions to refuse treatment
>
> – Lasting Power of Attorney (a legal document that allows people to state in writing who they want to make certain decisions for them if they cannot make them for themselves, including decisions about personal health and welfare)
>
> – a Preferred Place of Care Plan (which allows people to record decisions about future care choices and the place where the person would like to die)."

Indeed, as speech and language therapists we are in a good position to provide informational and counselling on these topics. We can encourage patients to consider their plans for the future, and empower them to voice their opinions about their own future care. Bourgeois and Hickey (2009) elaborate on this and suggest using advance directives in dementia care as communication tools to assist the person with dementia in structuring communication around care plans and treatment options.

In summary

Speech and language therapists have an important role to play in issues surrounding capacity. Advance directives and enduring power of attorneys are important methods for our patients to be confident that they will have their opinions heard as their dementia progresses. People with dementia have the right to make decisions around their own medical treatment, their finances and their living situation. If the people working with that person have concerns about that person's capacity to make these decisions then this needs to be assessed before it is assumed that the person lacks capacity. Speech and language therapists may then be involved in both facilitating the assessment to ensure the person with dementia is able to communicate (to the best of their abilities) as well as conducting such an assessment alongside another colleague.

Capacity assessment is increasingly becoming a core responsibility for speech and language therapists working with adults with communication difficulties. Consequently, we need to equip ourselves to be comfortable in this area. We have the knowledge and skills to understand the needs of people with dementia. The Mental Capacity Act can provide us with the knowledge around legislation and consequently the confidence to support our role as assessors and facilitators in this area.

References

Beauchamp, T.L. & Childress, J.F. (2001) *Principles in Biomedical Ethics*, 5th Edition. New York: Oxford University Press.

Bellhouse, J., Holland, A., Clare, I., & Gunn, M. (2001) Decision-making capacity in adults: Its assessment in clinical practice. *Advances in Psychiatric Treatment* 7, 294–301.

Bourgeois, M.S. & Hickey, E.M. (2009) *Dementia: From Diagnosis to Management – A Functional Approach*. New York: Psychology Press.

Department of Health (2005) Mental Capacity Act (2005). London: Department of Health. http://www.legislation.gov.uk/ukpga/2005/9/contents

Cameron, L. & Murphy, J. (2006) Obtaining consent to participate in research: The issues involved in including people with a range of learning and communication disabilities. *British Journal of Learning Disabilities* 35, 113–120.

Diener, B.L. & Bischof- Roasario, J.A. (2004) Determining decision-making capacity in individuals with severe communication impairments after stroke: The role of augmentative-alternative communication (AAC). *Topics in Stroke Rehabilitation* 11(1), 84–88.

Dreer, L.E., Devivo, M.J., Novack, T.A., & Marson, D.C. (2012) Financial capacity following traumatic brain injury: A six month longitudinal study. *Rehabil. psychol.* 57(1), 5–12.

Flew, R. & Holly, C. (2011) Has the mental capacity act changed the way SLTs work? Conference Presentation at RCSLT Wales Board Professional Development Day: Best Practice in Delegation.

Griffith, H.R., Belue, K., Sicola, A., Kryzywanski, S., Zamrini, E., Harrell, L., & Marson, D.C. (2003) Impaired financial abilities in mild cognitive impairment: A direct assessment approach. *Neurology* 60(3), 449–457.

Henson, A., Gildertson, Z., Azzopardi, P., & Pope, L. (2012) Talking rights: Communication access and mental health law. Poster Presentation. British Aphasiology Therapy Symposium, 6–7 September 2012, City University London.

Kirshner, K.L., Stocking, C., Wagner, L.B., Foye, S.J., & Siegler, M. (2001) Ethical issues identified by rehabilitation clinicians. *Archives of Physical Medical Rehabilitation* **82**(2), S2–8.

Lo, B. (1990) Assessing decision-making capacity. *Law, Medicine and Health Care* **18**, 193–201.

Marson, D.C., Stephen, J.D., Sawrie, M., Snyder, S., McInturff, B., Stalvey, T., Boothe, A., Aldridge, T., Chatterjee, A., & Harrell, L.E. (2000) Assessing financial capacity in patients with Alzheimer disease. A conceptual model and prototype instrument. *Arch. Neurol.* **57**(6), 877–884.

Moye, J. & Marson, D.C. (2007) Assessment of decision-making capacity in older adults: An emerging area of practice and research. New Directions in Aging Research, *Journal of Gerontology* **62**b(1), 3–11.

Moye, J., Karel, M.J.M., Azar, A.R., & Guerrera, R.J. (2004) Capacity to consent to treatment: Empirical comparison of three instruments in older adults with and without dementia. *The Gerentologist* **44**(2), 166–175.

Murphy, J., Gray, C.M., & Cox, S. (2007) How 'Talking Mats' can help people with dementia to express themselves: Full report. Joseph Rowntree Foundation. Downloaded from: http://www.jrf.org.uk/sites/files/jrf/2128-talking-mats-dementia.pdf

Murphy, J., Oliver, T.M., & Cox, S. (2010) Talking Mats and involvement in decision making for people with dementia and family carers: Full Report. Joseph Rowntree Foundation. Downloaded from: http://www.jrf.org.uk/sites/files/jrf/Talking-Mats-and-decision-making-full.pdf

National Collaborating Centre for Mental Health commissioned by the Social Care Institute for Excellence National Institute for Health and Clinical Excellence (revised 2011) THE NICE -SCIE GUIDELINE ON SUPPORTING PEOPLE WITH DEMENTIA AND THEIR CARERS IN HEALTH AND SOCIAL CARE. National Clinical Practice Guideline Number 42 published by The British Psychological Society and Gaskell. Downloaded from: http://www.nice.org.uk/nicemedia/live/10998/30320/30320.pdf

Royal College of Speech and Language Therapists (2005) Speech and language therapy provision for people with dementia. RCSLT Position Paper. London: RCSLT. Downloaded from: www.rcslt.org/resources/publications

Skinner, R., Joiner, C., Chesters, L., Bates, L., & Scrivener, L. (2010) Demystifying the process? A multidisciplinary approach to assessing capacity for adults with a learning disability. *British Journal of Learning Disabilities* **39**, 92–97.

8 Measuring outcomes of therapy

As mentioned in Chapter 1, The Department of Health in the UK released its White Paper titled 'Equality and Excellence: Liberating the NHS' in July 2010. In this document a system of GP commissioning was proposed. The White Paper outlines that "GPs coordinate all services that patients receive, helping them navigate the system". Consequently, the GPs are "best placed to coordinate commissioning of care for their patients". This White Paper does highlight the crucial role GPs already hold in managing long-term conditions such as dementia. Their proposal for this change in commissioning structures, such that the GP will be coordinating the commissioning of services including speech and language therapy, suggests that we may need to change the way we work to guarantee future funding for our services. Indeed, the Alzheimer's society warns that although this type of local decision making (by GPs) could support local services it may equally increase the risk of the postcode lottery in service provision.

Commissioning of services is often driven by outcomes. In general practice, speech and language therapists typically do collect some kind of measure of therapy outcomes. However, at present there is no real agreement amongst clinicians as to the most useful outcome measures for people with dementia. What is clear is that goal setting and patient or carer feedback are some of the most commonly used, and most sensitive, measures for this population. Equipping ourselves with evidence-based care pathways for patients, accompanied by clear outcome measures, will reduce the risk of patchy service provision for speech and language therapy services in dementia care.

This chapter addresses some of the key issues we have highlighted earlier, including goal setting and patient- or carer-reported outcomes.

Outcome measures for dementia

The UK's Department of Health published the document 'Living Well with Dementia: A National Dementia Strategy' in 2009. In this document, they highlight that people with dementia in general hospitals have worse outcomes in terms of length of admission, mortality and institutionalization than other patients. These types of measures provide little information on the effectiveness of interventions such as speech and language therapy. The report also highlights that general hospitals are particularly difficult for people with memory and communication difficulties, with cluttered ward layouts, poor signage and other hazards. These may be areas we as speech and language therapists can influence, but how can we demonstrate that any change has made an impact on someone's experience?

Can we show the people who commission our services that we provide some value for money as a speech and language therapy service and consequently ensure that they will continue commissioning our services? RCSLT (2009) make it clear that "Value for money is not about being the cheapest option but about delivering the most return (impact, best outcomes) for a given investment over time". And, ultimately, services provided to people with dementia should aim to impact on and enhance their lives in some way, be it their actual physical health or their quality of life. This emphasizes the need to ask patients for their opinions about what they perceive to have been the outcome of their care and the impact on their quality of life (Bourgeois & Hickey, 2009; Murphy, Gray & Cox, 2007).

What measure to use and why?

Choosing the most appropriate outcome measurement tools for patients with dementia can be very tricky, as for any progressively deteriorating disease (Kindell & Griffths, in Bryan & Maxim, 2006). In fact, there is very little research that examines the effectiveness of speech and language therapy with dementia (Bryan et al., 2006). This means there is no clear evidence about which path to choose when we are trying to decide how best to evaluate the effectiveness of our services. (See Table 8.1 for a brief description of outcome measurement for dementia and speech and language therapy.) There are also very few recommendations in this area of practice. The Scottish government did publish a document called 'Realizing Potential: An Action Plan for Allied Health Professionals in Mental Health' (2010) where they recommended that "Allied Health Professionals should use information gathered while providing interventions to evaluate the service user experience, enhance the evidence base and improve services using patient-reported outcome measures and standardised assessments".

In practice, however, goal setting and patient or carer feedback are some of the most commonly used, and most sensitive measures, for this population. Goal setting can be helpful in demonstrating to a patient exactly where their areas of communication needs are and how these have changed through therapy, therefore assisting to increase their insight and understanding of their condition. Goal setting can also highlight that therapy has achieved what was initially agreed, thus providing motivation and satisfaction. Similarly, this approach can be helpful to record the gains being made in therapy, so illustrating if therapy should continue or when an individual may be ready for discharge. Patient and carer feedback can also ensure that patients have an opportunity to indicate their satisfaction or dissatisfaction with the service they have received. See Chapter 3 for a more detailed discussion on how to set goals with a patient; Table 8.2 also describes three particular approaches to goal setting for people with dementia.

Table 8.1 Brief description of outcome measurement for dementia and speech and language therapy.

Method of measurement	Brief description
Assessment Formal or standardized measurements and Functional Measures – see Chapter 2: Assessment	Therapy outcomes should be specific to the target behaviour being addressed in therapy, and so should measure the frequency and magnitude of these behaviours. Use of standardized impairment-based measures in dementia would not be valid as outcome measures as it is not reasonable to expect changes on a such a test when the treatment goal aims to modify a specific behaviour (Bourgeois & Hickey, 2009). Having said that, there are some approaches to assessment (particularly non-standardized, more functional assessments), such as conversation analysis, that prove useful if the therapy being carried out aims to improve effectiveness of conversation between that particular dyad. Indeed, functional tests have better validity than impairment-orientated tools as they address the everyday needs of a patient with dementia (Bourgeois & Hickey, 2009).

(Continued overleaf)

Rating scales TOMS / AUSTOMS	Rating scales are often designed specifically to demonstrate outcomes of therapy. They are sensitive to functional changes in behaviour and are easily comparable with other services. However, many of these tools have not been designed specifically with the dementia client group in mind, so clinicians need to be careful to choose a tool that is sensitive to the effects of their therapy with this client group. Currently, there is no real agreement about which tools best suit people with dementia in speech and language therapy. In discussions in clinical forums speech and language therapists often report using rating scales such as TOMS or AUSTOMS with people with dementia (Psychogeriatric Special Interest Groups, 2012). This may be most useful to reflect maintenance of skills.
Goal -based outcomes (see Table 8.2 for further details on goal setting) Care Aims Model Goal Attainment Scaling Patient Related Outcome Measures (PROMS)	Many authors emphasize the value of using goals as an outcome measure with people with dementia, e.g. Ramsey, Heritage & Bryan, 2006; Bourgeois & Hickey, 2009). Bourgeois & Hickey (2009) emphasize that goals set with patients with dementia should be functional and measurable, and should clearly specify a functional skill or behaviour that will be targeted. Goal-setting measures do demonstrate that therapy has achieved what it said it would, and have the additional benefit of acting to facilitate the process of review and discharge (Bryan & Maxim, 2006). However, using goal setting can limit your ability to compare client groups and services. Efforts have been made to formalize the goal-setting process in order to address this. This is reflected in tools such as Goal Attainment Scaling.
Patient/carer reports: East Kent Outcome measurement Scale (Johnson, 1997). Patient Related Outcome Measures (PROMS) Questionnaires	Patient and carer questionnaires can capture perceptions of change in a patient's functional skills following intervention (Ramsey et al., 2006) as well as their satisfaction with services. They are perhaps the most sensitive of the measures, but also the most vulnerable to bias. Speech and language therapists often report using informal measures designed by their own service, or modified versions of Patient Related Outcomes Measures and the East Coast Outcome Measures with client groups with dementia (Psychogeriatric SIG, 2012).

Table 8.2 Description of goal-setting approaches that have been used with people with dementia.

Care aims	Kindell and Griffiths (in Bryan &Maxim, 2006) suggest using the Care Aims Model for goal setting as a way of capturing the breadth of the speech and language therapist's role when working with people with dementia. The Care Aims model is a way of "describing, measuring and representing" what a speech and language therapy service provides using eight categories of care (Malcomess, 2001). Care aims can facilitate collaborative goal setting by ensuring clarity about the purpose of intervention. It focuses on reducing the risk and the impact of a problem. The eight categories describe the aims of intervention, thus measuring clinical effectiveness according to what the focus of care is, not whether the condition has necessarily changed (Malcomess, 2001). Each episode of care can be measured by reviewing the goals set in each area. This demonstrates whether care aims have been achieved and can be used to monitor performance. The eight categories of care outlined in Care Aims are as follows: • assessment (identifying problems and potential for change) • rehabilitation (improving and lasting change) • curative (resolving problems) • enabling (maximizing current function) • supportive (supporting to optimal level) • maintenance (maintaining and preserving function) • anticipatory (preventative) • palliative (pain relief and comfort)
GAS	Goal Attainment Scaling (GAS) consists of a 6-step process. The patient or caregiver is invited to participate in an interview with a clinician to identify areas of difficulty or 'problems', and consequently identify goals for those areas (often consulting with the multidisciplinary team before these are confirmed). The next step is weighting the goals from most to least importance. A follow-up time is decided and finally the expected outcome is discussed, i.e. type of change. By identifying all potential levels of attainment (e.g. what would be better than expected, or worse than expected) the team is able to score outcomes specifically. The expected outcome is labelled as a '0' whilst less than expected may be scored as −2, or −1, and better than expected as +2 or +1. Finally, the baseline level is documented, i.e. the patient's status at time of writing goals. At the previously identified follow-up date, the goals are reviewed and the patient is scored on the level they have attained. These scores can be inserted into a formula that can calculate total outcome from all goals set. Bouwens, van Heugten & Verhey (2008) describe how the Goal Attainment Scaling (GAS) tool allows for both individualization of goals according to the needs of each patient as well as standardization of measurement by using a summary formula that calculates the extent to which a patient's goals are met.

(Continued overleaf)

Patient Related Outcome Measures (PROMS)	The Scottish government recommend that allied health professionals should use PROMS to monitor patient experiences both on entering a service at the assessment stage and on exiting the service. Reid (2012) describes using PROMS as an outcome-focused conversation using talking points at the start and end of therapy intervention. She explains that talking points focus on the person's aspirations and engages them in identifying what is important and what they would like to change. This approach also assists patients and staff to plan and record outcomes so that they can be measured. Reid (2012) found that patients with dementia were able to communicate what they needed from therapy and later identify what actually helped them achieve this such as 'being listened to' and 'having a say'.

What does the evidence tell us?

Outcome measures should not only be responsive to change, reliable and valid but also be tailored to the personal goals and needs of patients and their caregivers in relation to their daily life (Bouwens et al., 2008). Yet, as previously mentioned, there is little to nothing in the literature on outcome measures that can be applied to speech and language therapy for people with dementia.

Rating scales are often quick and accessible once you are familiar with them, and measures such as the AUSTOMS tool are useful approaches for patients being seen on an individual basis for maintenance therapy. However, there is no specific research that I am aware of that has validated the use of AUSTOMS specifically for people with dementia. Other rating scales are more appropriate for different interventions, so tools such as the Pragmatics Profile might be best used for therapies targeting social skills training, but again there is no real research into the use of this tool with patients with dementia. Bryan and Maxim (2006) describe using a modified version of the East Kent Outcome Measures Scales (Johnson, 1997) with patients with dementia. They report that this model allowed them to work with both patients and carers to ensure that expectations of therapy were realistic and specific areas of concern could be addressed. The information on patient-reported outcome measures is also still in its infancy and the next stage is to consider how best to use data being gathered (Reid, 2012). Similarly, care aims have only really been described anecdotally in clinical magazines or briefly in books. In fact, there is still some discussion as to whether care aims are a useful outcome measure (Bulletin, December 2012). However, Goal Attainment Scaling is somewhat more established and there is some more research that we can look to in this area, examining its use with people with dementia.

Bouwens et al. (2008) conducted a literary search of all studies that examined the feasibility of Goal Attainment Scaling (GAS) with the psychogeriatric population to explore the applicability of this tool for the dementia population. They examined a total of 10 studies that matched their search criteria. Bouwens et al. (2008) found that nine of these studies were from the same centre. Although this poses a limitation to the study it could also act as an indicator, suggesting that others have found negative results which have led them not to publish data or simply that this approach is under-used. Yet the authors of this review felt that that GAS is a sensitive measure for older adults with both cognitive and physical limitations. And furthermore, GAS can take into account features of dementia such as its progressive nature that many other measures cannot account for.

Bouwens et al. (2008) do highlight there are limitations to using the GAS tool with people with dementia. They describe how difficult it can be to engage individuals with dementia in the conversation required for setting goals with the GAS. They also explain that patients with dementia frequently lack insight into their impairments and difficulties. However, the studies suggest that using carers or modifying presentation methods such as using a goals menu can support this process. Another significant limitation of this tool is the time required to complete it. However, Bouwens et al. (2008) advocate strongly that GAS provides a lot of relevant information that otherwise remains hidden when multidisciplinary approaches are used. In fact, they state: "GAS is a unique example of an instrument able to reflect the multidimensionality of dementia and other psychogeriatric conditions, including interference with daily life activities, for both patient and caregiver".

At present there is no single measure for speech and language therapists working with people with dementia that is obviously better than others. Yet goal setting approaches and some patient-reported measures are leading the way as reliable methods of reflecting the positive impact speech and language therapy can have on peoples lives.

Other methods of measuring outcomes: Value-based outcomes

Ultimately, outcomes are the health results that matter for a patient's condition over their episode of care. This might mean that the most important outcome of an episode of care results in a slowing in the deterioration of the person's communication skills. Alternatively, an episode of care may result in increased functional independence and consequently less support required in their daily lives. In contrast to outcomes of care are the costs of care. This includes the total cost of care over that episode for that person. The difference between the two (health outcomes and total cost) is the 'value' of that care (Porter, 2012). He proposes that improving outcomes (quality improvement) should be the goal for improving healthcare (Porter, 2009). This will in turn reduce costs and improve value for money. He also proposes that the better your reputation for providing good care, the more patients will be referred to you, the more experience your service will gain, enabling you to collect more data that demonstrates your value and potentially increase the funding you may get to develop your service. Porter suggests that this is the cycle required to achieve high value care.

Porter (2009) emphasizes that understanding outcomes is about gathering data from outcomes measures but also on the total cost of patients' care. Cost of a patient's care encompasses all the actual resources that have been employed over the full cycle of their care including time (face-to-face time, note writing, etc), capacity (i.e. staff available) and support (i.e. resources such as training of staff, etc).

So perhaps it is less important at this stage to ruminate over which measure is best suited to the population we work with, but better to ensure we are collecting data on care costs as well as outcomes so we can demonstrate to commissioners the value provided by speech and language therapists working with people with dementia (see Table 8.3 for a example of what this might mean).

Table 8.3 Example of how to apply value-based outcome measures.

In Chapter 1 we asked the question:
Can you demonstrate the added value of speech and language therapy to the assessment process for the team and patient in a memory or dementia clinic?
Here is a suggested answer:
Setting up a pilot project can be a good method of trialling a change and can demonstrate the value of further investment into such a service. This might mean setting out an initial proposal, which outlines the costs of your resources (assessment tools, computer access, room space, administration support (paper, etc, staffing and supervision) to assess 20 consecutive patients being assessed by a memory clinic. To measure the effectiveness of this service you could consider the following:
• Questionnaires to staff before and after pilot
• Number of changes in clinical diagnosis and any other consequent changes in health management approaches, e.g. were they referred for therapy/recommended different medications
• Questionnaires to patients and relatives pre- and post-assessment and advice
• 3-month reviews of family after advice given

> By comparing the outcomes of these measures to the cost of your services you can demonstrate the value of your service. This pilot would hopefully demonstrate that both staff and patients/relatives value the extra assessment and advice you provide; you may also find that your added expertise provides additional information in making more accurate diagnosis (thereby perhaps reducing financial and health costs, ensuring accurate medications are prescribed and patients and relatives are able to use recommended strategies thus improving communication confidence and reducing carer burden).
>
> This may lead to more permanent funding arrangements as your reputation and value is established within the service. Clinicians will likely continue to refer patients for assessment and you can continue to demonstrate the value of this service. As your service grows you may also find opportunities to trial further therapy intervention such as therapy for patients with primary progressive aphasia.

In summary

With the current changes in commissioning structures within the NHS, we need to be even more aware of the need to demonstrate the value of our services. This may be through the use of widely-used outcome scales, goal setting or patient feedback. Focusing on concrete outcomes will help provide evidence for the value for money we can provide as speech and language therapists. Outcome measures can also support and guide clinical services to streamline the processes of admission and discharge.

References

Alzheimer's Society website (2012) Downloaded from: http://www.alzheimers.org.uk/site/scripts/news_category.php?categoryID=200288

Bourgeois, M.S. & Hickey, E.M. (2009) *Dementia: From Diagnosis to Management – A Functional Approach*. New York: Psychology Press.

Bouwens, S.F.M., van Heugten, C.M., & Verhey, F.R.J. (2008) Review of goal attainment scaling as a useful outcome measure in psychogeriatric patients with cognitive disorders. *Dementia and Geriatric Cognitive Disorders* **26**, 528–540.

Bryan, K. & Maxim, J. (2006) *Communication Disability in the Dementias*. London: Whurr.

Department of Health (2009) *Living Well with Dementia: A National Dementia Strategy*. London: Department of Health. Downloaded from: http://www.dh.gov.uk/prod_consum_dh/groups/dh_digitalassets/@dh/@en/documents/digitalasset/dh_094051.pdf

Department of Health (2010) *Equity and Excellence: Liberating the NHS*. London: Department of Health. Downloaded from: http://www.dh.gov.uk/prod_consum_dh/groups/dh_digitalassets/@dh/@en/@ps/documents/digitalasset/dh_117352.pdf

Johnson, M. (1997) Outcome measurement: Towards an interdisciplinary approach. *British Journal of Therapy and Rehabilitation* **4**(9), 472–477.

Kindell, J. & Griffiths, H. (2006) Speech and language therapy intervention for people with Alzheimer's disease. In K. Bryan, & J. Maxim (Eds) *Communication Disability in the Dementias*. London: Whurr.

Malcomess K (2001) The reason for care. RCSLT *Bulletin* **595**, November: 12.

Murphy, J., Gray, C.M., & Cox, S. (2007) How 'Talking Mats' can help people with dementia to express themselves: Full report. Joseph Rowntree Foundation. Downloaded from: http://www.jrf.org.uk/sites/files/jrf/2128-talking-mats-dementia.pdf

Porter, M.E. (2009) A strategy for health care reform – toward a value-based system. *The New England Journal of Medicine* **361**(12), 109–112.

Porter, M.E. (2012) Value based care delivery. Plenary session slides, Value Based Health Care and Value In Mental Health Event. London, England. February 29, 2012. http://www.uclpartners.com/lotus/wp-content/uploads/2012/03/20120229-Michael-Porter.pdf

Psychogeriatric Special Interest Group (2012) Psychiatry of Old Age Study Day (Southern UK).

Ramsey, V., Heritage, M., & Bryan, K. (2006) Developing speech and language therapy services in older age mental health. In K. Bryan & J. Maxim (Eds) *Communication Disability in the Dementias*. London: Whurr.

Reid, J. (2012) Talking about outcomes and dementia using talking points to promote meaningful engagement demonstrates the impact of allied health professionals' interventions. *Dementia AHP Approaches* **12**(1.2). Downloaded from: http://www.knowledge.scot.nhs.uk/media/CLT/ResourceUploads/4018744/DementiaAHPproachesSeptember%202012.pdf

Royal College of Speech and Language Therapists (2009) *Resource Manual for Commissioning and Planning Services for SLCN Dementia*. Downloaded from: www.rcslt.org/resources/publications

Scottish Government (2010) Realising potential: An action plan for AHPs in mental health. Downloaded from: http://www.scotland.gov.uk/Resource/Doc/314891/0100066.pdf

9 Finishing touches: Maintenance, review and discharge

What is considered best practice is not always best for the patient. What works for a patient does not always fit with commissioning and service models. Balancing best practice, patient needs and service level practicalities is part of our daily responsibilities. But this skill does not necessarily become any easier with experience. There are always new challenges, changes and developments to consider. Caseload management and discharge are often frustrating aspects of our role whether we feel we are managing it well or not.

This is a long and complex discussion and this chapter only touches the tip of the iceberg for some of these topics. However, we discuss what is currently considered 'best practice' in managing review and discharge for patients with dementia.

Review and maintenance

Patients with progressive conditions such as dementia will need input from speech and language therapy off and on throughout the course of their disease. But this does not mean these patients should remain on our caseload for the course of their disease. Bryan and Maxim (2006) stress that "typically intervention peaks and troughs alongside the patient and carers' journey".

Some authors such as Taylor, Kingma, Croot and Nickels (2009) and Duffy and McNeil (2008) advocate for regular review of patients with dementia. They highlight that communication and swallowing needs may change as the disease progresses and express their concern that later symptoms of dementia can include dysphagia. Bryan and Maxim (2006) are more specific and identify the following reasons to review a patient with dementia:

- to modify communication if changes are happening

- to assess if previous advice has been actioned or maintained or if any problems have arisen with specific advice given
- to address patient or carer stress and support
- to address care or care home environments.

However, Bryan and Maxim (2006) emphasize the important role of the wider team in managing patients with dementia. They highlight that, whilst one team member may discharge a patient, another – such as the nurse specialist or the GP in the community, and the nursing staff in a facility – might remain involved. There are also charities or other organizations that can provide social support and advice. Those staff that remain involved can act as the gateway to re-refer patients or encourage patients to seek re-referral should they require it, rather than clinicians having to continue reviewing patients indefinitely.

Our role as speech and language therapists is to empower patients living with chronic diseases and their families to be independent, managing their disease and seeking re-referral when they require it. This approach allows patients to make more independent decisions about when they feel they need advice, or are able to take advice and is much more in line with recommendations from NICE-SCIE (2011) who state that "people with dementia should have their voice heard in person centered care planning and reviews".

In short, speech and language therapy cannot continue indefinitely. Patients may benefit from a review if this is in line with their treatment – for example, to problem solve any concerns that have arisen with advice given at a previous session – but should be discharged once they have achieved their goals. On discharge, the process of re-referral must be carefully explained to a patient, particularly the reasons that might trigger a re-referral.

Case Study 1: Mr K

Mr K was a gentleman who was first referred to outpatient speech and language therapy by the movement disorders consistant with a recent diagnosis of Parkinson's disease and occasional swallowing and saliva management issues. His swallow was assessed and advice given. It was also noted at these appointments that he presented with a mild dysarthria. Consequently, he attended a series of appointments engaging in therapy addressing his dysarthria. Mr K was discharged from the speech and language therapy service, with the understanding he could seek re-referral via his

> GP or nurse specialist. Around nine months later Mr K was re-referred to speech and language therapy by his nurse specialist who reported concerns associated with further deterioration in his speech. During the nine-month period that he had not been to speech and language therapy he had been diagnosed with progressive supranulear palsy (PSP). At this appointment he also presented with word-finding difficulties and changes in his cognitive communication. He again attended for a series of therapy sessions and was discharged. Unfortunately, Mr K deteriorated further and was re-referred to speech and language therapy around a year later with further deterioration in his communication and changes in his swallow function. The speech and language therapist visited Mr K at home to assess his swallow function and support Mr and Mrs K in developing further communication strategies and developing communication aids.

When is maintenance therapy appropriate?

The use of the term 'maintenance therapy' can often cause concern for managers and therapists alike, as it infers that patients may have to attend therapy indefinitely to ensure their skills are maintained. But what does maintenance therapy really mean? Maintenance therapy is a programme that has been set up with the aim of stimulating the patient's language and communication to ensure the minimal amount of deterioration possible, i.e. to stave off the progressive process. In some ways, all intervention targeting language and communication for patients with dementia may be considered maintenance therapy. However, Bourgeois and Hickey (2009) emphasize that functional maintenance programmes are a way of providing a short period of intervention on a consultative basis. They describe this as a method of supporting carers around the patient or the patient themselves to implement a programme independently, which will work to maintain the person's communication skills at their best possible level once therapy has finished. They suggest that this may be recommended when patients appear to be plateauing in therapy and it is unlikely they will continue to improve. Bourgeois and Hickey (2009) hypothesize that this type of intervention may often be requested in a residential setting, but it is likely that more and more it will become part of the treatment planning involved for patients at the beginning and middle stages of their disease, especially for those living with the progressive aphasias.

Discharge

There is very little focus on how to discharge patients in the aphasia and general speech and language therapy literature (Hersh, 2009) let alone in the literature focusing on the dementias. Perhaps one of the most important things to say on this topic, however, is that discharge is important – particularly from the client's perspective. Indeed, Hersh (2009) emphasizes that "how we leave our clients at discharge can have a long-lasting effect".

In my experience, planning the process of discharge is easier the more transparent you can be with your patients. Indeed, commencing the discussion about discharge can start at the very first session you have with any patient, even a patient with dementia. This should involve coming to an agreement about what your goals are for therapy, approximately how many sessions may be required to achieve these goals and how often you will review your goals to check your progress. It is important to be clear that discharge is driven by goal achievement. Simply continuing treatment for people with dementia without such a plan may be futile (Tonkovich, 1999). Without a goal in sight, therapy has little value and may not enhance the quality of their communication skills. In fact, patients may prefer not to continue attending therapy.

Patients with progressive conditions such as dementia may actually decide that their priorities lie elsewhere, in managing or adjusting to other aspects of their condition. This might mean that therapy is not something they wish to pursue and will choose to discharge themselves sooner than you expect or feel comfortable with. Yet other patients may feel concerned about the idea of discharge. In these cases, it is worth remembering that there are services outside of the health sector that can also act as important links, particularly outside of periods of more intensive therapy, or on discharge (Bryan & Maxim, 2006). This can include charity organizations such as the Alzheimer's society and Dementia UK. It is not the speech and language therapist's role to provide ongoing adjustment counselling and emotional support. This may be much more effectively provided elsewhere.

When do we discharge a patient?

When therapists are asked about discharge from therapy they often report criteria such as "when a client plateaus, achieves their goals or when they are referred onwards" according to a survey of speech and language therapy services in Australia (Verna, Davidson & Rose, 2009).

The following are recommendations made by RCSLT (2006) and other authors (Bryan & Maxim, 2006) as reasons to discharge a patient:

- Intervention has finished and aims have been achieved
- Communication and swallowing are no longer a priority
- The patient and carer are satisfied
- Other team members will contact the speech and language therapist if required
- The patient is being transferred to another service
- The patient is able to self manage
- The patient is not compliant
- The patient has not attended and has been discharged as per local policy.

Due to the progression of the underlying disease process in dementia there may be a time when any therapy or treatment options are simply not reasonable (Duffy & McNeil, 2008). Croot, Nickels, Laurence and Manning (2009) highlight the importance of considering whether therapy is actually helpful for these patients; they remind us of the psycho-emotional distress that can be caused by participating in treatment. For example, by working on language skills the patient might be constantly reminded of how difficult this is for them. Be it grief, anxiety or personality changes that impact on these changes in coping, we must consider how this influences treatment and whether continued treatment is the priority at that time.

Case Study 2: Mr B

(See Chapter 4 for further information on this case study)

Mr B is a 59-year-old gentleman who was referred to the outpatient speech and language therapy service with a diagnosis of primary progressive aphasia of the semantic variant. Mr B attended all his appointments with his wife. They live quite a distance from the clinic and have to travel to the city, staying overnight the day before each of his appointments. Both Mr and Mrs B still work, and live at home with one of their two young adult children. Mr B attended outpatient speech and language therapy sessions on a weekly basis for almost eight weeks (see Chapter 4 for a summary of his speech and language therapy intervention). He decided to have a break from therapy and scheduled a review appointment for three months later. He then attended for a further six weeks of therapy, seeing both the speech and language therapist, the social worker and the psychologist. Mr B reported feeling increasingly 'depressed' about his diagnosis and that he disliked doing work outside of therapy sessions. Even attending therapy was depressing at times as it seemed to highlight all the things he couldn't do, yet when he was at work and out bowling (his current hobby) he felt he could forget about it and manage as well as ever. Mr B also reported having considered investigating options around selling their home so he could live more reclusively and not have to talk to people any more. Mr B's GP and geriatrician reviewed and modified his medications at this point, and he continued seeing a psychologist. At the end of this period, Mr B stated he did not wish to return to speech and language therapy in the near future as he wanted to focus on other aspects of his life. He suggested we start planning for discharge. At this point, Mrs B became quite concerned and sought advice and support from the social worker. As part of this process, Mr and Mrs B decided to appoint Mrs B as power of attorney for medical and financial decisions. Mrs B also got in touch with the Alzheimer's Society through which she made contact with other carers and relatives local to her. She found this a great source of support. Mr B continued to attend the specialist memory clinic based at the hospital every 3–6 months, and was advised he could seek re-referral to speech and language therapy through this service or through his GP.

How do we discharge a patient with dementia?

Having stated that speech and language therapists should ensure they do discharge patients (when appropriate), we need to consider how this is done. Discharge processes need to be carefully considered as they impact significantly on a patient's perception of therapy. Some research has been done to examine the impact of discharge processes on patients' perceptions of therapy in the stroke and aphasia literature. Hersh (2009) cites a study completed in the UK which reported that, following discharge after a period of rehabilitation, stroke patients and carers reported feeling 'abandoned by the system'. This suggests patients may be unlikely to return to 'the system' again. This would be an extremely negative outcome for patients with dementia, whom we would hope would return as difficulties progressed.

Specific research examining the experience of patients with aphasia after discharge highlights that these patients often do not even understand why they have been discharged (Hersh, 2009). They often feel that discharge is inevitable and they need to make way for other patients, not knowing if they can or should request more. In fact, some participants in this study described not wanting to be seen as difficult if they asked for more input. Hersh (2009) underlines that therapists need to participate more in discharge planning. This should dispel some of the myths around reasons for discharge and build a more positive relationship for future episodes of care. In doing so, Hersh suggests clinicians should ensure they do not overlook onward referrals to other services and long-term supports just because a person may appear 'happy' with discharge.

Research by Hersh (2009) does, however, describe some positive experiences in the process of discharge. The research highlighted that when decision making was shared, even if the person was not happy with the outcome of therapy, then they were satisfied with the process of discharge. Services that offered a gradual decline in therapy intensity were considered helpful in preparing patients, enabling them to get used to the idea of discharge. Similarly, services that offered follow-up were considered helpful in ensuring that patients did not feel abandoned. Patients reported feeling most able to cope emotionally with discharge if there were something else to occupy them (Hersh, 2009). We can learn from this report and use these strategies in managing discharge to ensure a more positive long-term relationship with our patients with dementia as they continue to dip in and out of our services.

The RCSLT (2006) guidelines reflect this evidence, and outline that the professional's duty at the time of discharge is to:

- Inform individuals of their re-referral routes and reasons
- Hand back care or hand over management of residual risks effectively
- Identify possible future risks and ways of managing these (particularly in the event that a patient has chosen to self-initiate discharge before the clinician feels they are ready).

These guidelines advise that part of the purpose of initial assessment is to open discussion with the person being treated or their carer about ultimate goals and discharge criteria, which will be reviewed and reconsidered through continued discussion throughout the intervention period. The RCLST (2006) guidelines also make recommendations about the use of a transition phase towards discharge, which allows the patient and therapist to agree a point of closure, and enables the therapist to support the individual through the process of ending therapy. They also recommend that the therapist should empower the individual to self-manage any needs that no longer require ongoing intervention from the speech and language therapist. Finally, RCSLT (2006) recommend that a discharge report be sent to both the patient and the patient's GP. This report should clearly state what the rationale was for discharge and provide guidance for re-referral procedures. This should ensure the patient and their GP are able to access information regarding re-referral in the future. Alternatively, including this type of information on therapy resources such as memory and communication aids can act as a constant reminder of your role. It may also facilitate easy access to your contact details in times of need.

In summary

Speech and language therapists need to consider carefully how they choose to manage patients with dementia in the long term, and be aware of all National Health Services as well as charity or independently-run organizations that are available to support patients and their families in the communities in which they live. Clinicians also need to spend time investing in the processes and plans for discharging their patients. Best practice guidelines in this area are well supported by studies that demonstrate which strategies work well from patients' perspectives in these situations. Endeavouring to discharge patients in a careful and considered manner can enable your department to ensure a more equitable service provision for all your patients.

References

Bourgeois, M.S. & Hickey, E.M. (2009) *Dementia: From diagnosis to management – A Functional Approach.* New York: Psychology Press.

Bryan, K. &Maxim, J. (2006) *Communication Disability in the Dementias.* London: Whurr.

Croot, K., Nickels, L., Laurence, F., & Manning, M. (2009) Impairment- and activity/participation-directed interventions in progressive language impairment: Clinical and theoretical issues. *Aphasiology* **23**(2), 125–160.

Duffy, J.R. & McNeil, M.R. (32008) Primary progressive apraxia of speech. In R. Chapey (Ed.) *Language Intervention Strategies for Aphasia*, 5th Ed. Baltimore: Williams and Wilkins.

Hersh, D. (2009) How do people with aphasia view their discharge from therapy? *Aphasiology* **23**(3), 331–350.

Kindell, J. & Griffiths, H. (2006) Speech and language therapy intervention for people with Alzheimer's disease. In K. Bryan & J. Maxim (Eds) Communication Disability in the Dementias. London: Whurr.

National Collaborating Centre for Mental Health commissioned by the Social Care Institute for Excellence National Institute for Health and Clinical Excellence (revised 2011) THE NICE -SCIE GUIDELINE ON SUPPORTING PEOPLE WITH DEMENTIA AND THEIR CARERS IN HEALTH AND SOCIAL CARE. National Clinical Practice Guideline Number 42 published by The British Psychological Society and Gaskell. Downloaded from: http://www.nice.org.uk/nicemedia/live/10998/30320/30320.pdf

Royal College of Speech and Language Therapists (2006) *Communicating Quality 3*. Downloaded from: www.rcslt.org/resources/publications

Tonkovich, J.D. (1999) Managing the long-term communication and memory consequences of dementia. *Neurophysiology and Neurogenic Speech and Language Newsletter* **9**(5), 9–14.

Verna, A., Davidson, B., & Rose, T. (2009) Speech-language pathology services for people with aphasia: A survey of current practice in Australia. *International Journal of Speech-Language Pathology* **11**(3), 191–205.

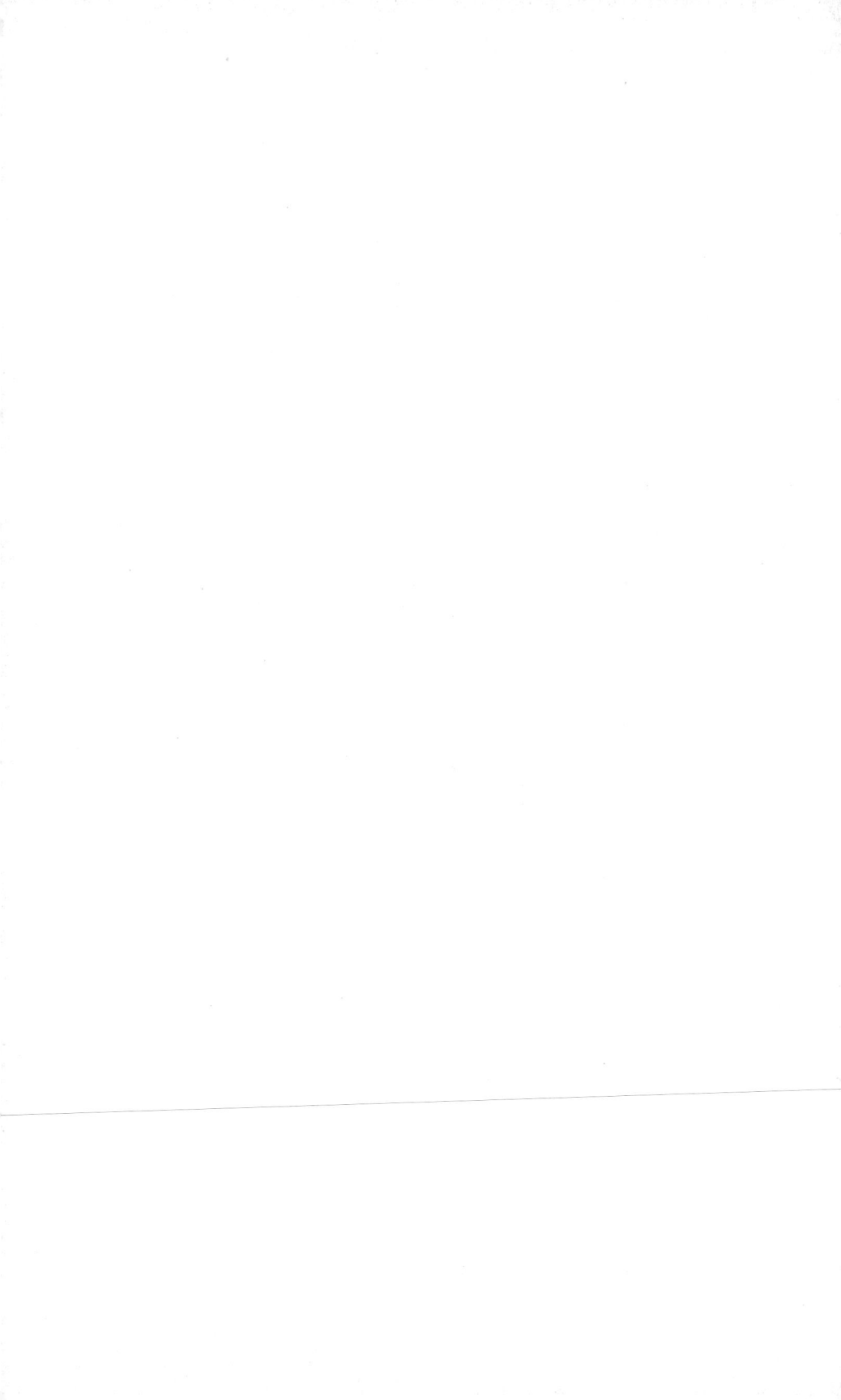

Afterword and useful contacts

People with dementia are seen on many different caseloads across physical and mental health settings, in acute, inpatient, outpatient and community settings. In 2013, NICE is publishing a new document entitled "Dementia: Supporting people to live well with dementia". This will be published as a NICE quality standard to stand alongside the NICE guidelines for dementia. It will be important to keep up-to-date with the most useful resources and therapy approaches because the area of health care for people with dementia is developing all the time. A list of useful contacts and websites to support you in keeping abreast of this information is given below..

Useful contacts for patients	Useful resource contacts for clinicians
Alzheimer's Society UK: www.alzheimers.org.uk	Pubmed search engine: www.ncbi.nlm.gov/pubmed
Alzheimer's disease International: www.alz.co.uk	NICE guidelines for dementia: www.nice.org.uk/nicemedia/pdf/CG042NICEguideline.pdf
Dementia UK and Admiral Nursing: www.dementiauk.org	Mental Capacity Act 2005: www.legislation.gov.uk/ukpga/2005/9/contents/enacted
The Frontotemporal Dementia Support Group: www.ftdsg.org	Access to useful new assessment tools for PPA: www.ftd-boston.org
Parkinson's UK: www.parkinsons.org.uk	Intensive interaction website: www.intensiveinteraction.co.uk
PSP Association: www.pspassociation.org.uk	SONAS aPc website: www.sonasapc.ie
MND Association: www.mndassociation.org	

Index

AAC (*see* Communication aids)
Activities and participation 19, 32, 120, 132
Adaptive interaction/intensive interaction 111, 117–119, 144, 150, 217
Advance decision/advance directives 168, 188–189, 192–195
Ageing 2–3, 30
Agrammatism 7, 22, 24–26, 29, 37, 90–91, 94, 96
AIDS/HIV 35–37, 46, 51
Alcohol 7–8, 34, 40
Alzheimer's dementia 6, 21–28, 30–34, 37–43, 45, 47–50, 78–79, 81, 85, 87, 90–91, 98–99, 114, 118, 126–127, 130, 135, 147, 154–155, 157, 161, 176–177, 180
Alzheimer's disease International 3-6, 15, 213
Alzheimer's society 3–5, 9,11,13, 32–35,124, 144, 152, 197, 210, 212, 213
American Speech-Language-Hearing Association (ASHA)   42, 45, 46, 47, 130
Assessment
  Case history 20, 38–41, 43, 51
  Conversation Analysis / Discourse 46, 48–51,145–150,199
  Formal assessment /informal assessment 35, 38–39, 42, 45–48, 50–51, 145–147, 171, 176–177, 199, 200
  Functional assessment 43–46, 48, 51, 181, 199–200
Aphasia, non-progressive 43, 44, 46, 66, 77, 82, 94, 99, 112, 147, 149, 210, 212, 212, 213
Apraxia 25, 29, 37
Arthritis 40, 175
Arizona Battery for Communication disorders (ABCD) 43, 47
Audiology 144
AUSTOMS 200,2 02

Binswangers disease 32
Boston Diagnostic Aphasia Examination 44, 49, 105
Boston Naming test (BNT) 44, 46
Burns Brief Inventory of Communication and Cognition 45
Barnes Language Assessment 45

Cancer 35, 40
Care aims 65, 200, 201, 203
Capacity assessment 167–196
  Consent to medical treatment 168–169, 171, 172–178, 180, 182, 183, 184, 185, 187–188, 191, 193

Finances 169, 179–180, 181, 185
Living situation 182–183, 186
Sexual consent 169, 186
Testamentary capacity 169, 186
Voting capacity 169, 186
Carers/caregivers (*see* Conversation partners)
Cognitive linguistic quick test (CLQT) 43, 51
Cognitive rehabilitation 110
Cognitive stimulation 66, 110, 136
Cognitive stimulation therapy (see groups) 119–120, 125-129, 136
Cognitive training 110
Commissioning 12–13, 197, 198, 205, 207
Communicating Activities of daily living (CADL) 45, 48, 113, 149
Communication aids 98–105, 115, 156, 173, 177, 187, 190, 209, 214
    Computers 82, 85, 86, 92, 95, 98, 99, 101, 103
    Talking mats (see Talking Mats) 98, 101–104, 187, 188–189
Communication Effectiveness Index (CETI) 113, 149
Communication passports 156, 159
Comprehensive aphasia test (CAT) 42, 43, 88
Computer-based therapies 82, 85, 86, 92, 95, 110, 130
Conversation Analysis (*see* assessment)
Conversation checklists 46
Conversation partners 5, 91, 12, 141–165
Cortical 24, 26, 32, 36, 37, 52, 81
Court of Protection 191, 192
Cueing techniques 77, 78, 79, 80, 92, 120

Decision making (*see* Capacity assessment)
Dementia,
    Incidence of 2–4, 12, 170
    Prevalence of 5
    Stages of 30–32, 62, 102, 113, 117, 131, 142, 176, 189, 209
    Variants of 5, 8, 10, 21, 29, 46, 90
Dementia with Lewy bodies 6, 7, 33
Depression 29, 37, 40, 63, 71, 96, 104, 127, 133
Deputy 181, 191–192
Diagnostic criteria 26, 83
Discharge 146, 168, 171, 182, 183, 184, 186, 188, 199, 200, 208–215
Discourse analysis (*see* Conversation analysis)
Downs Syndrome 7
Dysarthria 6, 32, 33, 34, 36, 37, 52, 159, 208
Dysexecutive impairment (*see* Executive skills) 37
Dysfluency 37
Dysphagia (*see also* Swallowing) 9, 11, 52, 174, 206
Dysphonia 37

East Kent Outcome Measurement Scale 200
Education 13, 19, 40, 52, 73, 141, 142, 143, 144, 148, 155, 156
    Group 119–124, 127, 143, 144, 150, 151, 155, 156
    Individual 111, 1 44
Empowerment 121
Executive skills 7, 109, 144

Fatigue 63, 157
FOCUSED program 150, 154, 158, 161
Fronto-temporal dementia 7, 13, 21–22, 26, 27, 121, 152, 180, 217
Functional assessment of communication skills for adults (ASHA FACS) 45, 113, 149
Functional
    Assessment (*see* Assessment)
    Intervention/therapy 51, 61, 63, 66, 70, 73, 79, 85, 95–96, 98, 100, 142
    Strategies 110
    Functional Linguistic Communication Inventory (FLCI)   45

Goal Attainment Scaling (GAS) 63, 65, 200, 201, 202
Goal setting 19, 38, 59–75, 93, 110, 112, 121, 123, 151, 160, 197, 199–205, 208, 210, 214
    Achievable 61–63
    Developing goals 68
    Examples of, goal setting 69–70
    Measurable 63–64
    Questions for 67
    Relevant 61

Grief 62, 72, 157, 211
Groups 119–136
    Combined exercise and communication 120
    Cognitive stimulation therapy   125–129, 134–135
    Conversation training (*see* Conversation training)
    Education (*see* Education)
    Reality orientation 119, 120, 125, 127
    Reminiscence 120, 129–131
    Sensory stimulation   132–134
    SONAS apc 120, 133–134
    Validation 131–132
    Support 13, 121, 123, 152, 155
Guardian 170, 187

HIV (*see* AIDS)
Holden Communication Scale 46
Huntington's disease 7, 21, 36
Intensive Interaction (*see* Adaptive interaction)

Korsakoff dementia 8, 34–35, 37, 78

Lasting Power of Attorney 168, 191, 194
Latrobe communication questionnaire 46, 145
Leaflets 144
Life review books 156, 158

Maintenance therapy (*see* Therapy)
Memory aids (*see* Communication aids)
External memory aids 113, 115, 158
Mental Capacity Act 167, 168, 173, 191,193, 195, 217
Mental Health Act 168, 184, 186
Mild Cognitive Impairment (MCI) 180
Mixed dementia 6
Motivation 61, 62, 63, 68, 71, 110, 158, 161, 199
Motor Neurone Disease (MND) 7, 28
Multiple Sclerosis (MS) 7, 21, 39
Multiple Systems Atrophy (MSA) 8

Naming (*see* Therapy)
Neuro psychology 20, 36, 39, 109
NICE guidelines 4, 9, 10, 11, 26, 122, 123, 125, 127, 136, 143, 152, 155, 156, 159, 161, 162, 168, 172, 194, 208
Non-fluent progressive aphasia (*see* PPA nonfluent/agrammatic variant)
Nursing home 12, 87, 96, 118, 128, 158, 162

Ophthalmology 144
Optometry 144
Orientation (*see* Reality orientation)
Orthographic lexicon 22, 98, 100
Outcome measures 64, 160, 162, 196–206

Patient centered 14, 46, 61, 70
Patient Related Outcome Measures (PROMS) 200, 202
Parkinson's disease/Parkinson's dementia 6, 7, 8, 33–34, 36, 37, 39, 40, 43, 51, 177, 208, 217
Peabody Picture Vocabulary Test 44
Phonological dyslexia 23, 99
Phonological loop disorder 25, 29
Power of attorney (*see* Lasting power of attorney)
Practice 63, 65, 71, 73, 81, 82–87, 92, 94, 100, 110, 160, 162
Pragmatics 33, 34, 36, 36, 111, 179
    Profile 46, 202
Primary Progressive Aphasia (PPA)
    Semantic variant 7, 22, 23–25, 26, 29, 37, 71, 78, 83, 84, 85, 87, 104, 141, 211

Index 223

Logopenic vvariant 7, 22, 24–25, 29, 90
Nonfluent / agrammatic variant 7, 22, 24, 25–26, 29, 85, 90, 94, 96
Progressive mixed aphasia (*see* PPA logopenic variant)
Progressive conduction aphasia (*see* PPA logopenic variant)
Progressive Supranuclear Palsy (PSP) 7, 26, 33–34, 52, 209, 217
Psychological factors 63
Psycholinguistic assessment of language processing in aphasia (PALPA)   44, 88
Pyramids and Palm trees test 44

Quality of life 10, 121, 126, 127, 156, 157, 198
Questionnaires (*see also* La Trobe Questionnaire) 12, 46, 112, 145, 162, 200, 204

REACH 155
Reading 23, 30, 38, 41, 42, 44, 45, 63, 67, 70, 78, 86, 87, 91, 92, 94, 98, 105, 109, 179, 181–182
    Therapy for (*see* Therapy)
Reality orientation (*see* Groups)
Relatives (*see* Carers)
Reminiscence (*see* Groups)
Repetition 25, 26, 29, 48, 51, 78, 79, 80, 85, 87, 187
Residential setting (*see* Nursing home)
Review (*see* Maintenance)
Rivermead Behavioural Memory Test   45
Royal College of Speech and Language Therapy (RCSLT)   10, 11, 14, 38, 60, 109, 156, 162, 171, 198, 211, 213, 214

Scripting (*see* Therapy)
Section 183, 186–287
Self efficacy 121–123
Semantic dementia (*see* PPA semantic variant)
Sensory stimulation (see Groups)
SIMS apc 111
Single words (*see* Therapy)
Small vessel disease 32
SONAS (*see* Groups)
Spaced retrieval 79, 80–81, 83, 85, 114.
Spelling (*see* Therapy)
Stroke 6, 11, 20, 21, 32, 38, 39, 43, 45, 51, 77, 78, 112, 175, 188, 212
Staff training (*see* Training)
Standardised test 27, 38, 43, 45, 46, 47, 48, 92, 131, 169, 198, 199, 201
Subcortical 32, 36, 37, 52
Supporting Partners of People with Aphasia in Relationships and Conversation (SPPARC) 51, 112, 144, 146, 148
Surface dyslexia 22, 29, 100, 103
Swallowing (*see also* Dysphagia) 8, 11, 34, 52, 175, 207, 208, 212

Talking mats 98, 101–104, 187–189
Teaching (*see* Training)
Television 51, 66, 69, 93, 95
Therapy
    Calendar management 81, 111, 114, 115, 116, 153
    Comprehension tasks 63, 77–89, 91, 92, 93, 95, 105, 135
    Gestures 91–92, 94, 101, 132, 152
    Maintenance 202, 209
    Naming 61, 63, 64, 73, 77–89, 104, 105, 114, 127, 135, 142
    Scripting 78, 90, 91, 92–96
    Self-monitoring 79, 87, 91, 92, 94, 109, 111, 144, 149
    Sentence 78, 85, 86, 87, 90–97, 99, 100, 109, 114, 136, 145, 150, 151, 152
    Single words 23, 24, 25, 29, 70, 77–89, 90, 91, 92, 94, 98, 99, 101, 104, 109
    Reading 63, 70, 78, 86–87, 91, 92, 94, 98–105, 109
    Role play 111, 186
    Spelling 98, 99, 100, 103
    Targets 62, 64, 70, 81–82, 94
    Verbs 78, 92, 94
    Video 82, 96, 104, 111, 112, 113, 146, 148–149
    Word finding 38, 83
    Writing 68, 70, 87, 92, 98–105, 109, 116, 141, 160
Thyroid dysfunction 40
TOMS (*see* AUSTOMS)
Topic maintenance 111, 112, 115, 145, 146, 147, 148
Training 10–11, 12, 13, 50, 73, 112, 113, 114, 115, 122, 141–165, 204
    Nursing staff 155–162
    Family 143–155
    Conversation training (*see* Conversation training)
Turn taking 111, 112, 113, 115, 117, 118, 145, 146, 147, 149

Validation (*see* Groups)
Value based outcomes   203–204
Vascular dementia 6, 32, 40, 114, 116, 124, 130, 175
Verbs (*see* Therapy)

Wernickes encephalopathy   34–35
Western Aphasia Battery   44
Word finding (*see* Therapy)
Writing (*see* Therapy)